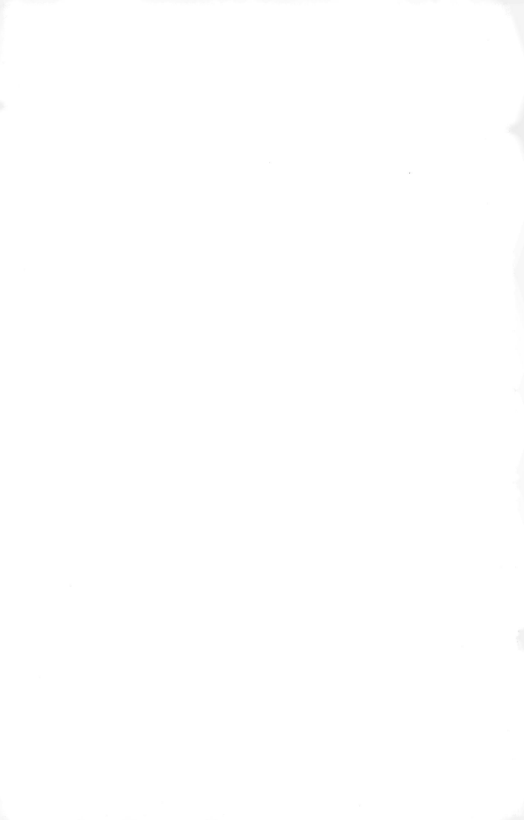

An Ethnography of Stress

Culture, Mind, and Society

The Book Series of the Society for Psychological Anthropology

The Society for Psychological Anthropology—a section of the American Anthropology Association—and Palgrave Macmillan dedicated to publishing innovative research in culture and psychology that illuminates the workings of the human mind within the social, cultural, and political contexts that shape thought, emotion, and experience. As anthropologists seek to bridge gaps between ideation and emotion or agency and structure and as psychologists, psychiatrists, and medical anthropologists search for ways to engage with cultural meaning and difference, this interdisciplinary terrain is more active than ever.

Series Editor

Rebecca J. Lester, Department of Anthropology, Washington University in St. Louis

Editorial Board

Linda Garro, Department of Anthropology, University of California, Los Angeles

Catherine Lutz, Department of Anthropology, University of North Carolina, Chapel Hill

Peggy Miller, Departments of Psychology and Speech Communication, University of Illinois, Urbana-Champaign

Robert Paul, Department of Anthropology, Emory University

Bradd Shore, Department of Anthropology, Emory University

Carol Worthman, Department of Anthropology, Emory University

Titles in the Series

Adrie Kusserow, *American Individualisms: Child Rearing and Social Class in Three Neighborhoods*

Naomi Quinn, editor, *Finding Culture in Talk: A Collection of Methods*

Anna Mansson McGinty, *Becoming Muslim: Western Women's Conversion to Islam*

Roy D'Andrade, *A Study of Personal and Cultural Values: American, Japanese, and Vietnamese*

Steven M. Parish, *Subjectivity and Suffering in American Culture: Possible Selves*

Elizabeth A. Throop, *Psychotherapy, American Culture, and Social Policy: Immoral Individualism*

Victoria Katherine Burbank, *An Ethnography of Stress: The Social Determinants of Health in Aboriginal Australia*

An Ethnography of Stress

The Social Determinants of Health in Aboriginal Australia

Victoria Katherine Burbank

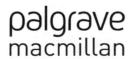

AN ETHNOGRAPHY OF STRESS
Copyright © Victoria Katherine Burbank, 2011.

First published in 2011 by
PALGRAVE MACMILLAN®
in the United States—a division of St. Martin's Press LLC,
175 Fifth Avenue, New York, NY 10010.

Where this book is distributed in the UK, Europe and the rest of the world,
this is by Palgrave Macmillan, a division of Macmillan Publishers Limited,
registered in England, company number 785998, of Houndmills,
Basingstoke, Hampshire RG21 6XS.

Palgrave Macmillan is the global academic imprint of the above companies
and has companies and representatives throughout the world.

Palgrave® and Macmillan® are registered trademarks in the United States,
the United Kingdom, Europe and other countries.

ISBN-13: 978-0-230-11022-9

Library of Congress Cataloging-in-Publication Data

Burbank, Victoria Katherine.
    An ethnography of stress : the social determinants of health in
aboriginal Australia / Victoria Katherine Burbank.
        p. cm.—(Culture, mind, society)
    ISBN 978-0-230-11022-9 (alk. paper)
    Includes bibliographical references and index.
        1. Health—Social aspects—Australia—Case studies. 2. Social
medicine—Australia—Case studies. 3. Indigenous people—Health
and hygiene—Australia—Case studies. 4. Stress (Psychology)—Social
aspects—Australia—Case studies. 5. Medical anthropology—
Australia—Case studies. I. Title.

RA418.3.A8B87 2011
362.10994—dc22   2010023205

A catalogue record of the book is available from the British Library.

Design by Newgen Imaging Systems (P) Ltd., Chennai, India.

First edition: February 2011

10 9 8 7 6 5 4 3 2 1

Transferred to Digital Printing 2011

Contents

Preface and Acknowledgments

The first thing, of course, is to survive . . .

—*Sahlins 2000:493*

When someone dies in an Australian Aboriginal community, people, usually, cease to use the name of the deceased from the moment they know of the death. In the remote Arnhem Land community of Numbulwar, the site of this ethnography, the deceased was often referred to as "body." One day when I was in the center of town, I heard a Council official announce on the town's loud speaker that "body comin'." Bodies often came to Numbulwar, usually from the Darwin hospital where people had been sent by health personnel in vain attempts to prolong their lives or with hopes that the severe medical conditions from which they suffered could be reversed. A background of ill health and death pervaded my fieldwork. There were constant reminders, the regular stream of bodies comin', the bodies I heard of between visits, often of people I had known since their youth, the days of "respect," and the weeks in which a body awaiting burial lay in the local mortuary. There were also the absences of people I had long known either because they were away for medical treatment, visiting another community to attend a funeral, or because they were dead. And these reminders insured that neither I nor others would spend a day, but rarely, without thinking and talking about our fellows' ill fortune.

I think of this book as an ethnography of stress. Both during the fieldwork and in this presentation of that material, I have been oriented by a social determinants of health framework. This framework draws our attention to social arrangements, particularly those generating social inequality and injustice that have physiological effects. A disturbing, but important, finding of this body of research is the long-term, even intergenerational, potential that social relationships have to harm. It is not simply the case that something like poor housing or poor diet causes ill health. The feeling that one is forced to inhabit an inferior house or eat an inferior diet may, in and of itself, makes us ill. It is feelings such as these that are increasingly seen as a kind of stress, and as I shall argue in these pages, these feelings must be always be regarded as in some way cultural.

I have had two sets of readers in mind as I have written *An Ethnography of Stress*. First is the group of anthropologists and students of anthropology who are largely unfamiliar with current developments in biology and psychology, and often wary of their use by psychological anthropologists like me. I hope that my extended and detailed treatment of what we generally regard as the cultural and the social via frameworks regarded as biological and psychological will persuade at least some readers that the integration of these distinct but highly relevant efforts greatly aids our attempts to comprehend our subject matter while circumventing both biological and cultural determinism.

My second imagined group of readers consists of people engaged in the study and practice of health, development, or some combination of these two fields, particularly those whose efforts have relevance for people who so far have been excluded from global prosperity. My intention in presenting a detailed ethnography is that it will act as something of a substitute for the years normally required to even begin understanding what life is like for people whose life experience diverges so dramatically from one's own. If this book enables greater well-being for the Indigenous people in Australia, I would be especially pleased, but I also hope that both the ethnographic material and the arguments I make about it may cast light on the predicaments of many disadvantaged groups.

Most of the material for this book was collected on three field-trips to Numbulwar, a remote Aboriginal community of about 800 people located in southeast Arnhem Land on the western shore of the Gulf of Carpentaria. Between 2003 and 2005, I spent about seven months there and another three weeks in Darwin, Northern Territory, where some people from Numbulwar live on a temporary or permanent basis. Over these months, I engaged in what anthropologists call "participant observation" or just plain "fieldwork". As the former term implies, I both observed and participated, insofar as I was able, in the life of the community.

Shortly after I arrived for my third and final field stint in 2005, I made the following journal entry:

> At least two strategies for living here. What I think of as the 9–5 crowd and the night life crowd. 9–5 have jobs, more education, live more by Western clock, more involved, e.g. jobs, with Western institutions. Night lifers sleep until late, stay up late, night probably long been

a way of escaping white gaze. These are drinkers, ganja folk, more likely living off unemployment vs. CDP [a form of welfare]. Younger people, perhaps, likely, more male than female. Christians would be 9–5. Not always clear cut divisions, e.g. card players in both. Re: well being, night life crowd may diminish this for 9–5 crowd, diverting money for gambling, drugs, alcohol, unnecessary? consumer goods. Making noise at night when 9–5 trying to sleep. Over burdening with childcare, hygiene, subsistence activity. (2005 I:49)

Most of the people I spent time with, and interviewed, would fit into the 9–5 crowd. But the night life crowd is not absent from these pages. As my journal entry indicates, these are not hard and fast categories. Some people with jobs may drink alcohol. Parents of school children, leading a 9–5 life, may nevertheless smoke, and even occasionally sell, *ganja*, that is, *cannabis*; those worried about their teenagers' drinking and smoking may once have sniffed petrol themselves. Christians who no longer drink, gamble, or smoke ganja may once have done so; an increasing number of Numbulwar's church population are just such people. People in the 9–5 group, especially younger ones, might well attend the discos and concerts that are occasionally held in this small town. They might also walk around after dark to meet friends or a lover. Almost everyone I know, except the most devout Christians, gambles in the seemingly ubiquitous card games held day and night. In addition, I can think of no family that does not include night lifers, if only because all families have numbers of younger people in them. Sadly, I can also think of no family that has not been touched by the kinds of trauma so pervasive in this community today: dysfunction, disease, and death.

During the three field trips, I spent my time visiting people but mostly being visited, shopping in the shop, picking up mail, and using the cash machine in the Council office, visiting the school and the community health clinic, arranging parties and meals for the Aboriginal family that has counted me among their number since my first trip to Numbulwar in 1977. Near sunset, I walked along the beach, tide permitting, exchanging a few words with children or groups of women as they returned from collecting pandanus leaves or mussels, noting in passing those fishing in the Gulf's channel and the motorized dinghies that might be returning with a dugong, a sea turtle, or the alcohol and cannabis obtained sometimes from Groote Eylandt just kilometers across the water. I also attended funerals, all that were held during my visits. These, of course, were funerals of kin. For the most part, however, my time and energy were devoted to conversation, particularly to doing the kind of careful listening my interests in person, psyche, and experience require. I was able to do a substantial amount of this although my time at Numbulwar was relatively short, no doubt because of my long association with the community and number of previous visits there.[1]

This work was supported by an Australian Research Council Discovery Grant (#DP0210203) received with Professor Robert Tonkinson and Dr. Myrna Tonkinson, titled "Inequality, Identity and Future Discounting: A Comparative Ethnographic Approach to Social Trauma." As the grant title implies, our intention is to write a comparative ethnography of Numbulwar and Jigalong—the Tonkinsons' principal research site for this study. To produce such a comparison, however, we first need to analyze and interpret our respective field materials. The results of these first analyses for Jigalong have appeared in a series of papers.[2] To present the bulk of my material on Numbulwar, I have written this book. Only in a text of this length have I felt able to contextualize the material in the manner I think it requires and begin to present readers with the details I deem necessary to understand my argument and my experience in this community.

Those who are up on Australian happenings will notice that the fieldwork for this book was collected before what is known as "the intervention," or the "Northern Territory National Emergency Response," a series of actions taken on the part of the conservative Australian federal government in 2007—the last year of its eleven years of power—as a response to reports of sexual abuse of children in Aboriginal communities in the Northern Territory. What effects it may have had on Numbulwar and how circumstances there may have changed since the time of the research are not clear. Phone conversations during the writing period suggested that besides a couple of community meetings with an intervention team and medical examinations for all children, little has occurred. A news item on the Australian Broadcasting Corporation's 7:30 Report, however, suggests that the intervention may not be off to a good start; a private company it contracted had "dug a pit toilet on a sacred site" at Numbulwar. "I been hurting myself inside because I saw this toilet," said one of the Aboriginal men interviewed. If such an event presages the kinds of changes that the intervention will bring, then, regrettably, this book will only become more pertinent.

Numbulwar began as the Rose River Mission in 1952. It has long been a relatively homogeneous community. The majority of people living there, with "country" contiguous to the settlement or nearby, derives from people who speak or once spoke Wubuy. These people may refer to themselves as Nunggubuyu, that is, "people who speak Wubuy" (Heath 1982:126). Others, such as those whose forbearers once spoke Ngandi, Ritharngu, Wanrdarang, Mara, and Anindiljuagwa are integrated into the community through decades, if not centuries, of intermarriage, shared ceremony, and shared history, particularly that of the Church Missionary Society's presence in the area.

I especially want to thank the Aboriginal people of Numbulwar who have shared so much of their lives, experience, and ideas with me over so many years and enabled me to become the kind of anthropologist I am. I also want to thank the whitefellas I have encountered at Numbulwar, who have, without notable exception, always been interested in and supportive of the work I do. I particularly appreciate the contributions from the whitefellas present at Numbulwar during this research period.

Ideas invariably develop over time, false starts made and corrected, seemingly incoherent arguments rendered intelligible, and blind spots hopefully filled. For help in this regard, I gratefully acknowledge Rita Armstrong, Bree Blakeman, Chris Birdsell-Jones, Chilla Bulbeck, Pat Draper, Zoran Grujic, Farida Iqbal, Chris Haynes, Emma Kowal, Julie Manville, and Warren Shapiro, my PhD supervisor of long ago who sometimes still supervises me. Being able to present an early version of chapter three to the Anthropology and Sociology Red Ink Collective enabled me to better understand and communicate with readers not so immersed in my theoretical framework, as did the opportunity to present this chapter at an Anthropology Seminar at the University of Sydney. I wish to thank Martin Forsey, Deborah McDougall, Laura Merla, Yasmine Musharbash, and Michael Pinches for their suggestions. I also wish to thank Jandran Mimica and Gaynor Macdonald for arranging the latter occasion and Ute Eickelkamp for providing me with a copy of the seminar questions and replies. Greg Acciaioli, Loretta Baldassar, David Butler, Richard Davis, Nick Harney, Gillian Hutcherson, Debra Judge, Jane Lancaster, Bev McNamara, and Maria Puerta Francos provided me with useful references when I was seeking literature in unfamiliar areas of study. I thank John Bern for his suggestions about historical sources and Carly Lane for presenting me with a copy of John Mercers' self-published book of children's stories based on his experiences in the earliest days of the Rose River Mission. Gill Hutcherson provided me with useful instruction on the finer points of English grammar. I appreciate David Trigger's comments on the original research proposal and on a paper "From bedtime to on time: Why many Aboriginal people don't especially like participating in Western institutions" (Burbank 2006) in which an important theme in this book first took form. I thank the Taylor and Francis Group for permission to use a substantial part of it in chapter six of this work. This paper was previously published in *Anthropological Forum* 16(1): 3–20 (http://www.informaworld.com). Some of the original content has been rewritten to better mesh with its new context.

The isolation required by writing, especially of an extended work, would not be tolerable without the engaged support of my fellow anthropologists here in Australia and abroad. In this regard, I would also like to thank Aleksandar Janca and John Laugharne, whose enthusiasm for my work was an important source of sustenance, as were the wise words of Aldrew Relph. Without the research assistance of Michaela Evans, Manonita Ghosh, and Bonita Wormsley, it would have taken me much longer than it has to write. I very much appreciate their enthusiastic and professional help.

My trips to the Northern Territory were more productive, comfortable, and fun than they might have been, thanks to Wendy Asche, Jane Balme, David and Lesley Mearns, Mick Reynolds, Kate Senior, and Ian White. I also wish to thank the Henry and Uibo families for decades of friendship and invaluable help.

Bob and Myrna Tonkinson and I have been together on this now for many years, as the research proposal developed and feelings and ideas resulting from the multiple field experiences sorted through. So too has Jim Chisholm, whose interests and ideas have long provided a stimulus for mine. The patience that all three have displayed, reading multiple drafts of this book, presents me with a shining example of academic generosity. Katie Glaskin kindly provided a second opinion on the revised conclusion.

Emily Buckland, Catie Gressier, and Jill Woodman have held the fort in Anthropology and Sociology at the University of Western Australia during the years I have written this book. All have provided greatly appreciated assistance on multiple fronts. Emily's maps at the beginning of this book and in chapter three must be mentioned in particular. I should also acknowledge a period of "Study Leave" from the University of Western Australia that provided me with some of the months used to write. I thank the editors of the Society for Psychological Anthropology's series *Culture, Mind and Society*, Professors Alexander Hinton and Rebecca Lester, for helping me through the submission and review process. I also thank the anonymous reviewers for their support and suggestions and the Palgrave

Macmillan editorial staff for helping me see this book in print. Last, but hardly least, I thank John Gordon for helping me find the additional time that I needed to finish this manuscript.

Notes

1. My first research trip to Numbulwar took place over eighteen months between 1977 and 1978, my second in 1980 lasted about nine months. In 1988 I returned, this time with James Chisholm and our then three-year-old son for a period of some seven months. Distance and family responsibilities kept me from returning to Numbulwar until 1997 when I was able to spend a brief but full five weeks there.
2. At the time of this writing, these include M. Tonkinson 2008, 2011, R. Tonkinson 2004, 2007a, 2007b, and M. Tonkinson and R. Tonkinson 2008.

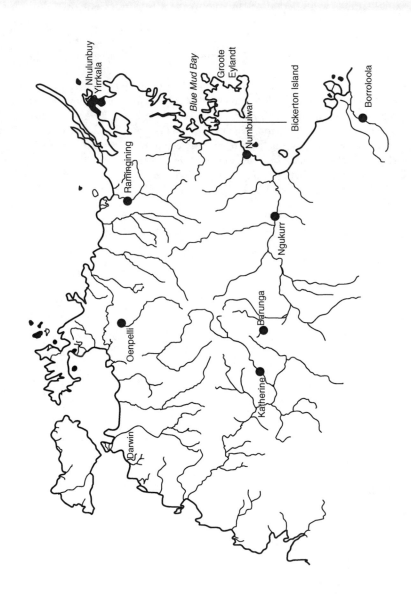

Nhulunbuy
Yirrkala

Blue Mud Bay

Groote
Eylandt

Bickerton Island

Borroloola

Numbulwar

Ramingining

Ngukurr

Barunga

Oenpelli

Katherine

Darwin

Chapter 1

Introduction: Using Social Determinants of Health, Using Ethnography

*Should we continue to do studies that arrive at forgone conclusions sim-
ply by exploiting the nonindependence of measures? (Such studies inevitably find that stress is generally bad, that perceiving relationships as
supportive is good, and that coping—though this is difficult to demonstrate—must be good.) Or should we undertake the much more difficult
task of identifying the complex and dynamic links among persons
experiencing recurrent periods of disruption and dysfunction in their
lives, how they lead their lives, and the nature of their social contexts?*

—Coyne and Downey 1991:403

In this book I "undertake the much more difficult task" set by Coyne
and Downey of "identifying the complex and dynamic links" among
life circumstances, experiences of stress, and their effects on lives
and circumstances. Focusing on Numbulwar, a remote Aboriginal
community in southeast Arnhem Land, Australia, my ethnographic
effort is framed by a "social determinants of health" perspective.

For some years now, both Indigenous and non-Indigenous
Australians have been observing, no doubt with varying degrees of
emotional intensity, disproportionate incidents of premature and pre-
ventable mortality in Indigenous communities across the continent.
Although Indigenous deaths may be underreported (Cunningham
and Paradies 2000:46), a routine finding of studies by such enti-
ties as the Australian Bureau of Statistics (ABS) is the existence of
a significant difference in the risk of mortality that falls out along
Indigenous/non-Indigenous lines. At the time this work began,
reports suggested that this difference in risk might be as great as 20
years, depending upon the design of the study (e.g., ABS 2003; Gray
et al. 2004; Zhao and Dempsey 2006). The ABS has published a

recent life expectancy estimate, for the years 2005–2007, arriving at the figures of 11.8 years for males and 10 for females, which might at first glance suggest a considerable narrowing of the mortality gap. However, it had employed a new method for arriving at the figures and has "strongly advised against any comparison" with earlier life expectancy estimates (ABS 2009:5). In any event, for the Northern Territory, the area within which Arnhem Land is located and hence of greatest relevance for this work, the differences continued much as before: for males this was 17.2 years and for females 13.4 (4–5).

At Numbulwar, people appear to be like Indigenous people across Australia, falling gravely ill and dying before their time.[1] The magnitude of severe illness and premature death—reducing the substantial number of years that people at Numbulwar are likely to live, or live reasonably healthy lives—must have a major impact on the families and community in which these lives are to be found. Thus, in this book I focus on the implications of premature morbidity and mortality at Numbulwar, on what may be, largely, but not exclusively, the sociocultural precursors and accompaniments of this state of affairs. These may be understood, at least initially, as stressful circumstances and experiences. In these pages, I present my attempt to understand something about them, including how they might have contributed to the ill health of people at Numbulwar.

Over the years, I have, along with many of my anthropological colleagues, come to accept that in our ethnographic efforts we do not describe sociocultural realities so much as interpret them (e.g., Geertz 1973; Marcus and Fisher 1986). And as we have come to accept this characterization of our activity, we have also come to accept the importance of our interpretive frameworks and of being conscious of them. It has become apparent that an understanding of anything is usually affected by prior understandings of something else, an insight derived from cognitive science, and schema theory in particular, from which the principal methods of this research are derived.[2] Confronted by the unknown and the unfamiliar, anthropological brains, just like any human brain, interpret new material via material already assimilated (e.g., Fernandez 1991). The important thing in ethnography is to do this with as much awareness as possible of the old material that is being used. My effort is, of course, framed and directed by my often unrecognized beliefs and expectations about humans in general, Aboriginal people in particular, and myself, as well as by the more formal theories and constructs from which I explicitly draw.

An identification of macrotropes in ethnography, that is, of tropes that "operate across the span of an entire ethnographic text" (Rumsey 2004:268–9), provides me with a means of both thinking about and foregrounding for readers the formative, but largely implicit, background assumptions that guide the ways in which I proceed in the field and subsequently present what I have learned from those efforts. Given my subject matter, it would be tempting to structure this book using the human body as a metaphorical device. Instead, what I have found emerging as I have thought about, written, and rewritten this text is better identified as an "ecological," or "body in a niche," metaphor, a metaphor that, perhaps not accidentally, has been used before in discussions of Indigenous health and stress in Australia (e.g., Beck 1985; Cawte 1978).

Doubtless, the presence of an ecological trope in this text arises from my engagement with a theoretical literature that emphasizes the integration of biological and cultural factors in contrast to, and in response to, what amounts to various versions of the nature/nurture debate.[3] Integrative approaches may be seen as arguments against the causal priority of materialism or idealism, the exclusion of culture from mind or mind from culture. These approaches emphatically counter arguments that present only what is labeled "culture" or "biology" as the predominant source of whatever human action or condition is under scrutiny. In contrast, and importantly in my view, integrative perspectives enable takes on the human condition that find cause yet eschew determinism, whether biological or cultural; they emphasize emergent outcomes and hence possibilities not intended and yet to be imagined. Simultaneously, integrative perspectives incorporate ideas of constraint without which is it difficult, if not impossible, to identify dysfunction, pathology, and injustice.

Appropriating these ideas, I have been able to work from the inside out, focusing on the person in the niche, as I do toward the end of this book when I explore the development, meaning, and experience of "Aboriginal identity" in chapter five and the development and implications of a "cultural self" in chapter six. I have also been able to work from the outside in, focusing on encompassing social, historical, and cultural environments in which I find Aboriginal persons. My treatment, in chapter three, of historical experiences as possible precursors of contemporary ill health is an example of this perspective. Juxtaposing both tacks, I am able to present a picture of past and current environments that suggest the "complex and dynamic links" contributing to people's ill health and premature death without implying that these are necessary or inevitable. Just as importantly, such integrative frameworks, arising as they often, if not always, do from a consideration of our species' evolutionary history, reinforce my insistence that this book not be read simply for information about an Indigenous Australian condition. Rather, it should be read to better apprehend, predict, and, it is hoped, circumvent some aspects of the human condition. Here we may regard with some apprehension the Aboriginal people of Numbulwar as an advance guard of the disadvantaged; many of us already suspect that we will not live out our lives in the relative material and psychological comfort of our parents' generation.

In the remainder of this introductory chapter, I discuss what is known as the "social determinants of health" perspective, a model, or perhaps more precisely a family of models, with similar features that provide the most immediate framework for this work. I also discuss, insofar as I am able to, the ways in which I work at Numbulwar and later, back on the university campus, with what I believe I have learned while living there.

Social Determinants of Health and the Indeterminacy of Stress

Ideas that encompassing social structures affect people's well-being are at least as old as Marx and Durkheim, weaving their threads though a century of scholarship and research (Mechanic 2007; Saggers and Gray 2007:5). Recently, however, we have been presented with what I see as a particularly promising perspective that helps us implicate and explain nonbiological factors in the genesis of ill health without dismissing the importance of biology. This is what has been labeled "the social determinants of health" model. Its beginnings may be found in the correlational studies of social epidemiology, initiated in large part by the work of Marmot and his coworkers (Marmot and Wilkinson 1999) at the International Centre for Health and Society at University College London. Also largely thanks to this work, we can conceptualize a "social gradient of health." The finding that inspired this concept best captures just what it represents: differential mortality rates were found to be inversely correlated with employment grade in the British Social Services, that is, men working in lower grades were, in stair-step fashion, more at risk of death from coronary heart disease than those in higher grades, even when major medical risk factors were held constant.[4] Thinking around this concept has led to considerations of the possible causal roles that rank and hierarchy might play in health status (Anderson 2007:23–4; Wilkinson 1996:64–5).

Attempts to identify and understand the mechanisms behind the social gradient—the specific biological and psychological processes that translate social disadvantage into ill health—are even more productive for a study such as mine. Building on Sapolsky's work (1993), Brunner and Marmot (1999) have described the human stress response, otherwise known as the "fight-or-flight" response (LeDoux 1996; Panksepp 1998), as the critical physiological pathway that leads from social environment to person in this regard. The ways that we manipulate our experiences of subordination to minimize or deny them and respond to experiences of relative as opposed to absolute poverty suggest that, along with other primates, we appear to not like being the "low man on the totem pole" (Sapolsky 2004:408,410). Feelings such as "anger," "fear," "exclusion," and "disappointment," to use English constructions of such feelings, may be read as manifestations of an activated stress system. This neurophysiological system, understood to be inherited in large part from our mammalian forbearers (Panksepp 1998), is thought to have been fine-tuned for human service by natural selection in environments, both physical and social, radically different from those we live in today. When it enables an organism's escape from a finite danger, it produces the physiological changes needed for fight-or-flight, and then returns to its resting state. When, however, the source of perceived threat is a more or less continuous one and when people experience a "lack of predictability" and "lack of control," have little or no means of understanding the sources of their distress or expressing their frustration with them, and when they receive little support in their social environment, then the stress system may remain engaged in a manner that can have major negative consequences for physical and mental health (Brunner and Marmot 1999; Sapolsky 2004:396–7).

It cannot be insignificant that the illnesses associated with an overactive stress system are more or less the same ones that have laid so many Indigenous people so low (Brunner and Marmot 1999; Condon et al. 2004:450; Cunningham and Paradies 2000:31–2; Zhao and Dempsey 2006). At Numbulwar, health clinic personnel implicate the "metabolic syndrome" as the preponderant source of adult ill health. Obesity, high blood pressure, and type 2 diabetes are the plague of many. Because the metabolic syndrome contributes to kidney failure and coronary heart disease, these conditions are not uncommon in the community. For example, over the three years of the field study, I knew of 10 people from Numbulwar who had left this community of about eight hundred for Darwin, where the dialysis they needed to stay alive is available. I also knew of one young man who had received a kidney transplant some time before the research. Of the people on dialysis during the study period, one now has a new kidney; three others died.

It remains, however, to identify and explicate the sources of stress in the lives of Indigenous Australians and their social and behavioral responses to them. While the beginnings of this effort are to be found in the collection *Social Determinants of Indigenous Health* (Carson et al. 2007) and the report of the Adelaide International Symposium, *An Overview of the Existing Knowledge on the Social Determinants of Indigenous Health and Well Being in Australia and New Zealand* (Pulver et al. 2007), these are early days in the application of this perspective to Indigenous health in Australia. As those who look at social determinants of health have noted, when we consider any social source as the cause of ill health, we must also consider the complexity of biological and environmental interactions, including such components as beliefs, feelings, and emotions (Nguyen and Peschard 2003:451) that can, I believe, exacerbate or ameliorate the stress potential of any circumstance we might encounter. While there may be some arrangements or events that any human would find subordinating, controlling, or otherwise diminishing, there are undoubtedly others that would evoke a variety of responses.

From the outset of this research, I have assumed that the identification of what we call "stress" in other people's lives must foreground a consideration of their experience, that is, how they understand and feel about the arrangements and events others might think of as stressful or benign (cf. Adelson 2008). "Experience," I understand, in turn, is something to be investigated at the level of the person, with person conceived of as both a biological and a psychological entity. Experience is what people have, in the sense of what they think and feel as they interact with their environment. I must emphasize here my assumption that a human environment is always a culturally apprehended one, understood largely through knowledge and belief acquired from others in the processes anthropologists call "socialization" and "acculturation." Working with assumptions such as these, psychological anthropology seems particularly well equipped to identify "complex and dynamic links among persons experiencing recurrent period of disruption and dysfunction in their lives" (Coyne and Downey 1991:403).

The location of culture as much in individual minds as in its social and material manifestations (Geertz 1973; Linger 1994) is consonant with frameworks connecting stress and health. It is the bodies, including the minds, of individual people that experience stress and may fall ill because of it. The beginnings of this ethnographic approach to stress might be found in D'Andrade's (1995) warning that an anthropology without "psychology is an anthropology with empty people" (234), a resuscitation of Goodenough's (1971) location of culture "in the minds and hearts" of those who learn and share it (19). Here I join anthropologists, especially those in the community of psychological anthropology, who have resisted an exclusive focus on public manifestations of culture. An example of this orientation is to be found in Linger's (1994) thought. Inspired by the cognitive linguistics of Reddy and Langacker, he defines culture as "ideas in people" (297), whose intersubjectivity is predicated on their ability to use symbols to evoke, rather than convey, the meaning that is in another's mind. Anthropologists do not, Shweder (1996:27) might add, need to get into another person's head; they do, however, need to learn mind reading. To again use Linger's (1994) words, the anthropological task is to "infer as best one can the subjective worlds of other people" (293), to construct "provisional formulations of another's subjective experience" (294). Drawing on ideas about "schema" recently adopted by cognitive anthropologists (D'Andrade 1995:122–49), and, in particular, the work of Strauss and Quinn (1994, 1997) whose heuristic use of schema theory provides the principal methodology of this work, I have attempted to incorporate a surer sense of the minds that learn and share culture into this ethnographic account. At the same time, the schema concept has provided me with a means of pursuing culture in minds (Shore 1996).

Schema theory presents any form of knowledge—whether about self, other, inanimate object, or abstract thought—as patterns of neural connection, formed via the process of associative learning. As a person interacts with the environment, existing schema are activated—and modified by previously unencountered or unattended components of the environment—as mental representations of both the regularities and novelties of the current experience (e.g., D'Andrade 1995; LeDoux 2002; Strauss and Quinn 1997). Depending upon the circumstances of learning, and circumstances may be internal as well as external, the neural substrate of experience may manifest as one image, idea, belief, and so on, or as a collection, which in turn may be more or less coherent. As neural connections once made are thought to be rarely if ever unmade, there is a component of permanence in any experience, including those of "identity" and "self," concepts central to this work to be discussed in later chapters. Schemas, however, do not prevent us from learning new things. Past residual may then become part of a new configuration and hence experienced as in some way different (Quinn 2006; Strauss and Quinn 1994, 1997). This new and somehow changed experience can include that of self or identity.

Via schema theory we can understand human communication, and culture, as the capacity to activate schemas in another person that represent experiences similar to our own. This activation is accomplished most efficiently, of course, via talk or other symbolic behavior. The idea of schema also allows us to see that although we may feel in perfect accord with another, as we do from time to time, we must nevertheless acknowledge that while understanding may be mutual, it is never identical. I can never claim to know exactly what my Aboriginal confidants think. Schema theory, however, encourages me to at least try to understand something of other people's experience. Symbols are not schema, but schema may be reconstructed via an analysis of symbols, in particular, those symbols we call words or talk or narrative or text. As decades of work in cognitive anthropology and related fields within psychological anthropology indicate, this is not easily accomplished (e.g., Quinn 2005a). In particular, as a "whitefella"[5] working in a remote Aboriginal community, I have found that eliciting the kinds of discourse that might contain clues to interior realities challenging, to say the least. Nor have I been able to tape record most conversations, a requirement for the highest standard of discourse analysis (Quinn 2005b:18–21). Nevertheless, I think I can offer a series of sketches that capture something of the understandings of Aboriginal people at Numbulwar during the study period.

My assumption that our environment is always a culturally apprehended one entails a further assumption, that there are culturally patterned as well as individual differences in the understanding and feeling of experience. And I recognize, of course, that when we face the possibility of culturally patterned difference we also face the problem of cross-cultural translation. An example of this kind of problem can be found in a comparative study of aging that included a Ju/'hoansi group in Botswana. For comparative purposes, people's responses to an interview protocol designed to access their perceptions of aging were collapsed into "higher level categories." But when Draper (2007), the anthropologist interviewing Ju/'hoansi, attempted to do so, she found she "could not readily distinguish between their answers that mentioned bodily strength and health and their answers that mentioned material well-being and material resources or 'wealth'" (683). Upon reflection, it occurred to her that "for the Ju/'hoansi their bodies were the same thing as their tools and wealth," that is, as hunter-gatherers it was as much with their bodies as with their tools that they obtained their living. Without this insight into Ju/'hoansi thinking, an account of their experiences of aging would have been impoverished, as would be our understanding of human aging more generally. During the course of the fieldwork and in the analysis of the material I have gathered, I have tried to remind myself that what I think is obvious may well not be for someone else, particularly for one whose experience departs from mine in significant ways (Sullivan 1970:20).[6] I make the case in this book that my acquaintance with those departures has been provided, at least to some extent, by the extended fieldwork I have undertaken at Numbulwar, not only for this study, but during the thirty-year time span over which I have been visiting this community. But before I begin to make this case, I think it best to introduce the reader to some aspects of my recent fieldwork at Numbulwar. Numbulwar as a sociocultural space will be the subject of the next two chapters.

Fieldwork at Numbulwar, 2003–2005

Journal entries

Wednesday, September 3, 2003, Numbulwar

Sept. 2 Arrived Numbulwar around 10:30 AM after 6:50 flight from Darwin–Gove, 8:10 MAF flight from Gove via Groote...Airstrip now has bitumen. Road to airstrip still unpaved with potholes and soft dust places...(2003:I:7)

Thursday September 4, 2003, Numbulwar

Around 10:10 Went to office and shop...Ran into Lily[7] and went with her to shop, new, on opposite side of road from old one which has been torn down except steel skeleton...Lily asks me when we are sitting [at a place] with [her son and daughter-in-law] what I'm here to do. I say to talk to people about how they are feeling these days about being Aboriginal people in Australia and about good and bad things here. Lily says things used to be good here. She has gone very grey. (2003:I:12,15)

Unlike my first fieldwork at Numbulwar, undertaken in 1977 and 1978, an effort that required every minute of the eighteen months I spent there, I was able to begin work within days after my arrival in 2003, though I had not visited the town for some years. From the start, I was able to hold substantial conversations with local people and participate with them in at least some of their daily activities. I was able to begin interviewing people within four weeks and during my visits in 2004 and 2005 within a week or two. In 2007, I visited Numbulwar for a week in February, not to do further research but to report back to the community upon the work so far.[8]

Shortly after my chance meeting with Lily, a woman who has assisted me on all of my visits (e.g., Burbank 1988, 1994), she agreed to help me phrase the questions I thought I might begin asking in the somewhat structured but open-ended interviews I conducted with twenty of Numbulwar's Aboriginal residents. Over the three years, these questions changed to some extent, depending upon answers I had received in previous interviews, and, of course, new questions arose as I spent more time living at Numbulwar and engaging in informal conversations with people there. I also interviewed eight whitefellas, men and women working at the town's office, homelands center, shop, school, and clinic. I interviewed eight Aboriginal people on at least two occasions, six of these numerous times across at least two of the study years. Two whitefellas provided me with interviews each year of the study. Most of the interviewees were women, only two Aboriginal people and three whitefellas were men. All were "adults," aged between eighteen and about sixty-five.

The interview questions I began with were derived from a central proposition of this research—that relatively new forms of self-identification, that is, the acceptance of an "Aboriginal identity," exacerbated stressful experience. This idea is not unlike questions that others have asked about the ways that ethnicity might contribute to ill health. In relation to substance abuse, Agar and Reisinger (2001) have looked at the kinds of historical circumstances that can change the ways an already marginalized people feel about themselves "from some previously 'normal' state of affairs" (740). The resulting "unresolved contradictions between expectation and reality" may increase "anger, frustration and depression among group members." Dressler et al. (2005) have proposed that the relationship between ethnicity and ill health may be understood via analyses of the ways in which culturally constructed identities enable or frustrate the achievement of valued goals (242). Some of those engaged in research on "subjective social status," understood as "the individual's perception of his own position in the social hierarchy" (Jackman and Jackman 1973 in Demakakos et al. 2008:331) while not addressing "ethnicity" per se, find that the social and economic resources that people have affect their evaluations of their social position. These evaluations, in turn, appear to have various effects on health (Demakakos et al. 2008:331).

The idea about "Aboriginal identity" resonating with my field experience at Numbulwar originated with Dr. Myrna Tonkinson, who has worked in the Aboriginal community of Jigalong in Western Australia since the 1970s. She thought that people's self-understanding as "hunter-gatherers" pursuing life as they knew it, encompassed, though not affected in any meaningful way by the surrounding Australian sociality, might have shifted to the invidious identity of "Aborigine." By this she meant a descendant of the original inhabitants of Australia, first invaded and then dominated by European settlers and regarded as inferior by many non-Indigenous Australians, even today. In this interpretation of her experience at Jigalong she was anticipated by Austin-Broos' (1996) discussion of "two laws" talk, Aboriginal discourse in which *blackfella* Law and *whitefella* law are juxtaposed, compared, contrasted and to some degree melded (4–5). Here Aboriginal people reflect on the processes by which their "primordial identity" becomes an "ethnicity," the form of identity that accompanies the "experience of difference that is also hierarchical" (6). Most germane to my study, however, was Tonkinson's idea that this new identity would affect Aboriginal people's sense of self and might also affect their sense of well-being. How to obtain evidence for or against this possibility that changes in identity were related to current states of ill health thus became the major task, and challenge, of my fieldwork. I also needed material that would allow me to identify the sources of stress that people at Numbulwar experienced.

Conversation was a central means of pursing both endeavors. This might be described as being of three kinds. The most conventional is the sort of conversation we think of when we hear the word, in this case, conversation between me and at least one other person. There were many of these over my three visits, as people visited me in my Health Department flat overlooking the Gulf of Carpentaria, as I visited people, rarely in their homes, more often at more public places such as the school or on the back veranda of the clinic, where health workers took breaks and visitors stopped by, or in chance encounters such as the one that Lily and I had near the shop on my first day out in the town. A second use of conversation I make is of that overheard, of children playing or quarrelling, of people passed by on the road or encountered in such places as the office or shop, or of those talking in a group of which I was an acknowledged part. A final source of conversation was that of the interview. Only on these occasions did I take notes during the conversation; these consisted of my questions and respondents' answers.[9]

Reading the texts to identify evidence of stressful experience in them came next.[10] Here, of course, I was faced with the expected imperfections of intersubjectivity, as human communication is sometimes grandly known. Everyone has likely experienced the slippages that occur in everyday social interaction when we attempt to transform the ideas of one person into the understanding of another. But beyond this, moving between Western academia and Indigenous remote community Australia, we enter into the realm of cultural difference and the necessity of cultural translation. I illustrate these issues with a discussion of how I interpret and use "emotion talk" (Abu-Lughod and Lutz 1990:14) to understand something of the experience of people at Numbulwar.

Using Emotion Talk to Approach Experiences of Stress

From its beginning as a named entity, stress has been linked with emotions. According to the psychologist Lazarus (1999), the origins of the "stress industry" are to be found in a concern with the consequences of war-related conditions, defined largely on the basis of emotional experiences such as "shell shock" and "post traumatic stress disorder" (28). The synonyms of the stress response, "flight" or "fight," are invariably associated with the English emotion terms of "fear" and "anger." Nor does contemporary neuroscience suggest that this link is inappropriate, though it clearly derives from folk theory. For example, the neuropsychologist Panksepp (1998) tells us that "the pituitary-adrenal stress response...accompanies virtually all emotions" (218), which is not to say that all emotions, or stress, are bad for us. In a review of the neurobiology and pharmacology of stress, pain, and opioids, Ribeiro et al. (2005) propose that emotions are one of the "common mechanisms that have evolved to deal with [environmental] stressors" (1265, 1266). Along with other forms of sensation, they "can be seen as closely connected to the preservation of homeostasis, contributing to the global representation of the physiological condition of the body and well being" (1265).

Emotions and pain are interconnected "to the feeling of homeo-static balance," that is, our sense of the extent to which there is a departure from homeostatic balance, otherwise known as our sense of stress. When pain becomes "encoded affectively and cognitively as an emotion" (ibid.), we do not experience it as pain per se. Our awareness of pain as the organic response to physical or psychologi-cal stress is not necessarily that of "feeling pain" but possibly that of just "feeling bad." That is to say, what we might come to experience psychologically as *fear* or *anger* or *stress* may originate as a neuro-physiological pain response (see also Eisenberger and Lierberman 2004).

Contemporary neuroscience also allows us to see ourselves as constantly feeling beings, a constancy that is seen by some work-ing within this area of scientific effort as coalescing in the "self" (e.g., Damasio 2003; Ribeiro et al 2005). It might be better, then, to speak not of specific emotions but of something like "core affect" (Russell 2003) as an ever-present part of our experience. It is curi-ous though that all languages surveyed in this regard have specific emotion terms, though not all of these languages have labeled an overarching category that may be translated "emotion" (Wierzbicka 1999). According to Russell (2003), this is "because people divide the world into categories" (160) and hence what he calls "emotional episodes" are categorized as a matter of course. I might even go fur-ther here and note Lakoff and Johnson's (1999) conclusion, based on a convergence of findings in the cognitive sciences, that we are compelled to categorize, given the bodies, brains, and external world that we have. Most of our categories are "formed automatically and unconsciously as a result of functioning in the world" (18). I assume that part of our functioning in the world includes functioning within our bodies, that is, that our functioning includes experiences of our-selves as feeling beings. The feelings or feeling complexes that we categorize with our culture's assistance become our emotions.

We also know from a fine collection of ethnography on emotions across space and time that people do not always form categories out of the same domains of feeling experience. From this work it has become apparent that we use English language emotion terms as scientific constructs at our peril. Such terms cannot, according to Wierzbicka (1999) and others, particularly Lutz (1985), provide us with a standard for cross-cultural comparison that does not incor-porate the implicit culturally specific theories, meanings, and values associated with these terms. These associations colonize the analysis, distorting our understandings of others' experiences. Also pertinent here are Reddy's (2001) ideas about "emotives"—emotion terms that both describe and alter our interior worlds—and specific cultural (or from another perspective historical) emotion regimes—"a normative order for emotions" (104–5, 124–6). It is from an emotion regime that we appropriate categories and practices arising from and evoking implicit theories, meanings, and values about people and the ways they feel. In particular, his argument that the emotion terms appropriated to explain our feelings to ourselves and others have the capacity to modify our feelings (see also Obeyesekere 1981, 1990) also signals the caution we need to take when attempting to portray and understand the kinds of cross-cultural experiences I write about in these pages.

We cannot, however, ignore Wierzbicka's (1999) finding that all of the diverse languages she has surveyed have terms she describes as "fear-like," "anger-like," and "shame-like" (286). She tells us that:

> All languages have words linking feelings with (i) the thought that "something bad can happen to me," (ii) the thought that "I want to do something," and (iii) the thought that "people can think something bad about me," that is words overlapping (though not identical) in meaning with the English words *afraid*, *angry*, and *ashamed*. (276)

These labels of experience, "fear," "anger," and "shame," are among those associated with stress by stress researchers:

> It should be obvious that certain emotions—for example, anger, envy, jealousy, anxiety, fright, guilt, shame and sadness—could be called *stress emotions*, because they usually arise from stressful, which refers to harmful, threatening, or challenging conditions. (Lazarus 1999:36)

Thus, Wierzbicka's finding points not only to the ubiquity of stress in human life but also to what may be a pan-human recognition that feelings arising from stress are worth categorizing, albeit that recognition might well be automatic and unconscious given the role that stress plays in the survival of all mammals, and undoubtedly once played for our hominid forbearers (LeDoux 1996).

Following decades of cross-linguistic comparison, Wierzbicka (1999) has concluded that while we need to be wary of the concept "emotion," another concept, rendered as "feel" in English, is available in any language. Feel has a universally shared meaning manifest in a sentence such as, "I feel like this" (16), a meaning, I suggest, that is shared because the vast majority of humans share the experience of bodily sensation. In her cross-cultural survey of feeling talk,

Wierzbicka has observed that "'ordinary people' generally assume that the way one feels can be described and that one can tell other people how one feels" (13). They may do so in three possible ways. They may describe themselves as feeling "good" or "bad," they may describe a scenario associated with a feeling, for example, "like something the dog dragged in," or they may give an account of the bodily sensations (such as blood beating in the temples) that co-occur with more cognitive feelings (such as those we call *anger*). Of course, people may use all of these strategies to describe any particular feeling.

As we can expect all people to talk about "feeling good" and "feeling bad," this provides me with considerable assurance that I can learn about and adequately, though not perfectly, represent at least some of the experiences that accompany activation of the fight-or-flight response for people at Numbulwar. Speaking of good and bad, Wierzbicka (1996) says: "These two concepts are innate and fundamental elements of human thought (experience can teach us to regard certain things as 'good' or 'bad,' but it cannot teach us the very concepts of 'good' and 'bad')" (52). Wierzbicka does not elaborate on what she means by "innate." While this is not the place for me to unravel her meaning, I would note the abundant evidence from divergent sources that many animals distinguishing what we label good from bad in the sense of "what is good for me," to be approached, from "what is bad for me," to be avoided or vanquished (Chisholm 1999:79–95). Indeed, according to Quartz (2003): "The capacity to approach nutritive stimuli and avoid aversive stimuli in the maintenance of life history functions is the hall mark of behavioral systems across phyla" (195). I find it unimaginable that such ideas are not included in the traditions of all human groups.

Furthermore, all of these terms—feeling, good, and bad—are, according to Wierzbicka (1996, 2005), English versions of conceptual universals; they are indefinable, that is, simply known, and have semantic equivalents in every language. For example, definitions in the Oxford Paperback Dictionary demonstrate the circularity that results when a semantic fundamental such as bad is defined:

> bad—wicked, evil
> wicked—morally bad
> evil—morally bad, wicked (Wierzbicka 1996:278)

The presence of *ambarlaman* and *aladi* in Nunggubuyu and *gud* or *guduon* and *nogud* or *noguduon* in Kriol, the two Indigenous languages most closely associated with Numbulwar, provide further support for Wierzbicka's nomination of good and bad as conceptual universals and add two more versions of them to her extensive cross-linguistic collection.

It seems reasonable to subsume harmful, threatening, and challenging circumstance under the concept bad, at least initially, and to begin my cross-cultural understanding of stress with Aboriginal discussions of "bad things." But I also need to ask if bad in Aboriginal English means the same thing that it does in the English I usually speak. It could be that other words and phrases—especially given the patois of Wubuy, Kriol, Aboriginal English, and English spoken to me at Numbulwar—are better translations of my word bad. This is where I see the usefulness of attending to scenarios and accounts of physical sensation. They help my running validation of intuitions that specific words and phrases mean what I think they mean. But I must also count empathy among my tools for cross-cultural translation.

In her book *Unnatural Emotions* (1988), Lutz discusses the use of the fieldworker's emotions to better understand and elucidate the emotional and social lives of people in other settings. Her concern to read both her own emotions and those of the people on Ifaluk according to their respective cultural scripts led to the use of her own feelings as a critical tool of discovery. For example, her surprise upon learning that *ker*, an emotion that might be translated as happiness, was regarded as "amoral, if not immoral" (44) enabled her understanding of *metague*, that is, roughly *anxiety/fear* as a moral emotion fostering conformity to the social order.

Though she disavows a complete dismissal of the psychobiology of human emotionality, Lutz casts emotions as "preeminently" cultural (5); emotion words provide "an index to a world of cultural premises and scenarios for social interaction" (210). Here emotions become cognitions in the commonsense meaning of the term, cognitions about self and social interaction. Thus it is not surprising that Lutz sets empathy aside, in favor of translation. Empathy is not particularly useful because emotions are not, as she puts it, "universal, natural and precultural" (42). She agrees with Rosaldo (1984) that the fieldworker can draw upon prior interpersonal, and by definition, emotional relationships, "to create a shared emotional understanding" (217). But empathy doesn't get us very far because emotions are really about relationships and "The ethnographer's position in the field would often seem to prevent the full development of the central conditions necessary for emotional understanding which is a shared social position, and hence a shared moral and emotional point of view" (217). Hollan and Throop (2008) remind us of a long-held anthropological suspicion of empathy as a research tool. I think, however, we should ask if Lutz was only thinking when she felt surprise. To my eyes she has clearly used her own feelings—an important step in evaluating the validity of one's resonance with another (Kirmayer 2008)—to great effect in producing what might be described as a "preeminently" empathetic treatment of emotional life on Ifaluk. Following her example, though counter to her methodological position, I count empathy as an important tool in my research, which is not, of course, to claim a perfect accord with any person at Numbulwar.

In a major Western philosophical tradition, empathy has been recast as *einfuhlung* (feeling into), "as a process of involuntary, inner imitation whereby a subject identifies through feeling with the movement of another body" (219). *Einfuhlung* is contrasted with *verstehen*, understanding. Understanding according to this contrast "is reflective, empathy is prereflective" (Makkreel 1995). I, however, prefer the definition of Fenichel in his work *The Psychoanalytic Theory of Neuroses* (1945): "Empathy consists of two acts: (a) an identification with the other person, and (b) an awareness of one's own feelings after the identification, and in this way an awareness of the object's feelings" (511). Recent neural imaging research indicates that entering into the thinking and feeling states of others—abilities most humans are believed to have from their early years, if not days, onward—draws on separate neural structures. Nevertheless, it is thought that an account of many empathetic experiences requires an account of both forms of brain activity—activity that in this literature is referred to respectively as "mentalizing" and "empathy"—as these activities are assumed to interact (Singer 2006). The greater accord of Fenichel's postulation of the near identity of thinking and feeling with current findings in neuroscience encourages me to think of empathy as the capacity to imagine/feel what another is feeling, yet know at the same time that one is not feeling what another is feeling. It also requires me to include translation as an inseparable part of an empathic ethnography.

One day, TeeJay, an adolescent girl, accompanied by her younger sister Brady, entered my flat with the words, "Auntie, I just threw up, because I'm not used to walking in the hot sun." Once seated, a glass of cold water at hand, she continued:

> Yesterday I got a phone call on my mobile, from [TeeJay's aunt] in Darwin. And I could hear near her [her husband] growling. He was angry. He want the truck, red one, got the bull catcher, gonna come

and pickem up, bring him back here to Numbulwar [probably for a funeral]. He was mad. He was saying he would call the police if they didn't come and pick him up. "Tell that girl staying in my house, my daughter, that's my brother passed away." And I went and told her. They've got the vehicle, but she said they had to get petrol, waiting for the barge to come in. [My uncle, auntie's husband] ran away from hospital, from dialysis. That doctor was looking for him and the police was looking for him. And [his brother] has something inside, his leg is swelling up and he is there in Darwin for dialysis too. Those two ran away. I growl at my uncles, I tell them not to drink grog, it is bad for them, making them no good inside. I growl at my uncles because I respect them. I like them. I don't want them to drink grog. My uncle called your [my fictive] sister three times, he wants to come back. He is driving her mad. And you know [TeeJay's adult cousin], he is cranky. I was playing video and Brady was playing the video at the house today and your [fictive] son was sitting, staring at us and he took the coke we bought at the shop and took three tablet, small one, and he drank the medicine, overdose. And then he walked to the beach and we watched him go. I don't like to see him. I don't like to see his face. I feel frighten and sad. I don't like to see him up close, only from a long way. He was growling, he was telling us he was going to ask [a third uncle] for $20 for ganja [cannabis]. I was growling at him, not to get ganja. He was talking bad word to his mother last night. And this morning he turned on the stove in our house. We were all sleeping; he tried to burn down the house. And my father and mother saw the smoke and my father put the red button on the power box and turned off the switch. And we saw your [fictive] son walking. And my father said he was going to belt him someday when he made him angry. When [TeeJay's uncle in Darwin] was angry and growling, he make me angry and I was growling back to him. And that Ben [another of TeeJay's adult cousins] is here at Numbulwar. He is supposed to be at Groote, for 10 months probation; if he is good behaviour he can come back here. He is supposed to be on Groote. You know [Groote man], he called my father on my mobile. He told him that the police are looking for Ben. He better go back to Groote. [A classificatory father] is going to send him back Friday. Police are coming here Friday. [Ben's wife] called my mother on my mobile three times last night because Ben went to her and was humbug [pestering that can take an aggressive turn] for ganja. He was on the hill yelling and swearing at her and she told me when she heard his voice she was frighten. He's not allowed to go near her. He's not allowed to touch [approach] that house for her. She has another husband now. (2004:V:22–5)[11]

Teejay's mobile phone seems to have acted as a lightning rod for attracting accounts of family trouble. The calls from her aunt, her uncle yelling in the background, the warnings from a neighboring community, and from a cousin's wife brought the immediacy of male anger and aggression to her, reminders of the extent to which alcohol and drug abuse, illness, and domestic violence plague her family. The phone also effected the heated verbal exchange with her intoxicated uncle.

Telecommunication, however, may merely have intensified her awareness of family problems. The cousin who almost burned down her house was right there staring at her while she and her sister played a video game. She could hear him swearing at his mother and watch him take what was probably psychotropic medication, possibly in excess, then walk off in search of cannabis in spite of her entreaties not to do so.

Did TeeJay find these events as disturbing as I might, had they happened in my family? In relating them, she makes use of scenarios that help me understand what she means when she uses words such as *mad*, *frighten*, *sad*, and *angry*, and so to judge the extent to which her experience might match what I imagine about mine. Her uncle is *mad* because he wants to return to Numbulwar, has been asking people to help him return to Numbulwar, and they are not doing so. He is "driving" his wife *mad* because he keeps calling her and telling her what he wants, which happens to be something his wife has little power to do anything about. TeeJay feels *frighten* and *sad* when an adult kinsman, her "cousin," stares at her, speaks aggressively, takes drugs, and either deliberately or accidentally almost burns down her house. People can make her feel *angry* when they speak aggressively and when she feels *angry* she speaks aggressively in turn. Understanding something of these scenarios makes me think I understand what TeeJay means when she says *mad*, *frighten*, *sad*, and *angry*. I also think that this, admittedly partial, understanding arises from my ability to empathize with her, not simply to think about but also to feel what it would be like to be in her circumstances.

This, however, is just the beginning of translation and understanding. To replicate something more of TeeJay's feeling experience I need to know more about the scenarios she presents along with labels for feelings; I need to know more about their cultural and biographical elements. For example, while the relationship between a mother's brother (i.e., "uncle") and sister's child is normatively one of mutual protection, nurturing, and discipline, a consideration of relative age would also likely be a part of the scenario. I might wonder here, if a part of this unmarried teenager's feelings about her uncle's actions would be the thought that while her reaction of anger and didactic aggression is appropriate, it was being required of her prematurely, that is, while she was still a schoolgirl. Similarly, I might note that a "cousin" may be an appropriate marriage partner if not regarded as "too close." However, the cousin staring at this teenage speaker is a very close cousin and staring is understood to be not only a sign of aggressive intent but also of sexual interest. There is much more of this nature to be said, but by adding just this small amount of further content to the scenarios I can imagine feelings that might go considerably beyond my experiences of *angry* and *frighten* and *sad*. Vomiting suggests that TeeJay was deeply, and noxiously, affected by this series of events. *Angry, frighten*, and *sad* are her words, but in my initial apprehension of them they do not capture all that she seemed to be feeling. When I use words, including emotion terms, that are not those used by people at Numbulwar in portrayals of their experience, I do so to offer, via my attempts at empathetic understanding including knowledge of the scenario, the best translation I can of what I think people are experiencing.[12]

Beyond its use in my discussion of empathy and translation, TeeJay's text is important for at least two other reasons. With some changes in detail, it could be an account of experience from anyone living at Numbulwar, or, I suspect, in any other remote community in Indigenous Australia. It also provides an extended example of the ways that people at Numbulwar talked to me, and to others, about their feelings, and the feelings of others, especially with regard to what might easily be identified as "harmful, threatening or challenging circumstances." I present accounts of these circumstances and how they appear to affect the lives and health of people in the chapters to follow.

In the next chapter, I focus on aspects of the research setting that are of particular relevance to this work. This introduction is necessarily just that, a sketch of the complex physical, social, and cultural environments in which I have long found the Aboriginal people of Numbulwar leading their lives. In highlighting the divergent experiences of blackfellas and whitefellas, the importance of relationships and family for Aboriginal people, and the likelihood of different value hierarchies that may be distinguished along blackfella and whitefella lines, I identify what I believe to be critical background material necessary for understanding the argument of this book.

Chapter 2

At Numbulwar: Blackfellas and Whitefellas

An Intercultural Setting

Numbulwar may be one of the most remote Indigenous communities in Australia. It has, since its establishment as Rose River Mission in 1952, been buffered, to a considerable extent, from settler culture by distance and a terrain of mangrove, eucalypt forest, bog, and sand not easily traversed, even on foot (Eastwell 1976; Thomson 1983). Distance, however, does not mean complete isolation from the encompassing Australian nation-state. Anglican missionaries from the Church Missionary Society were present from the beginning; Northern Territory Department of Education teachers have long staffed the school. The town's administrators, police, electricians, mechanics, plumbers, accountants, shop managers, pilots, doctors, and nurses, along with its school teachers, have always come from the larger Australian society, as have much of the town's physical infrastructure, its policies, rules, and other social arrangements. Radios, videos, music cassettes, and television, augmented by CDs and the Internet[1] in recent years, have been available there at least since the early 1980s. Though the vast majority of Numbulwar's population is Aboriginal, it might be said that "Western culture" has long suffused daily life.

From the perspective of at least some of Numbulwar's non-Indigenous residents, however, the local Aboriginal people were, during the study years, of "a different culture":

> I am [a man's fictive] brother...they treat me like a full family member but in the end they understand I'm from a different culture, so whatever. And it's the same thing for me. (UTG 2005)

> [A man], he's the one who walks around yelling about his [kinsman who died of heart disease before the age of 30]. I don't think though

that it really has that much to do with his [kinsman]. If he's stopped
to think a bit he's realizing that nothing good is ever going to happen
to him. If they sit down and think about what life is for them, they
are out of their culture and it's impossible to get into white culture.
I was thinking about this while hearing him yell today. It's so sad.
There is not enough of their culture left to sustain them, but there is
nothing else for them either. (TOT 2004)

He said, "When I tell you about this, you have to trust me." This was
when he was cutting [two men's hair] because he has to be careful,
what he does with the hair. Because someone could do something
with his hair. [One of the men] said this. That's why [this man] was
coming in and having his hair cut, and he, more than probably anyone here, he's so very experienced in both cultures. And he was worried. Children talk about [sorcery], especially unexplained deaths,
where it's young people. (ITU 2005)

A big problem is that this is still a group of people under control
of whites. They have to succumb to white rules and regulations, a
white way of life. They don't have control. There is no self determina-
tion on a community. The structure of the Council, it's a whitefellas"
structure, with minutes, the way of talking. They don't talk like us,
so what are they doing in that environment? It's that attitude and
climate that these people have to conform to white ways. There is a
lot of strength in their culture that overrides monthly Council meetings but most in the larger world would say that's a major problem.
(BIM 2003)

While the word "culture" had entered the language of both whitefellas and blackfellas at Numbulwar by the time of this study,
for decades now anthropologists have been asking themselves
whether or not the concept, once so central to the anthropological endeavor, is of much use (e.g., Abu-Lughod 1991; Trouillot
2003). Generally, they agree that culture is "learned" and, to varying degrees, "shared"; there is less agreement about just what it is,
where it might be located, and what if anything it does (e.g., Boyer
1993; Geertz 1973; Goodenough 1971; Keesing 1974; Linger 1994;
Spiro 1951). Nevertheless, a concern on the part of ethnographers of
Indigenous Australia to depict the forms of sociality and experience
that have emerged from sustained interaction between Indigenous
and non-Indigenous people has led to conceptualizations of the
"intercultural" (Hinkson and Smith 2005), a term recently rein-
troduced to Australianists in the work of Merlan (1998).[2] She has
described "an 'intercultural' account as one which attempts to deal
with the relations among different forms of experience, knowing
and practice" (2005:174).

To exemplify what such an account might be, Merlan (2005) draws on the experience of Julie, an Aboriginal woman living in the town of Katherine,[3] who tells her about the time when road workers dug up a small rainbow serpent (167). Julie understands that the road workers were improving the road, but having told her mother that the road workers dug up something, and having her mother explain to her that this was a young rainbow serpent, she has experienced things in a way that varies from what we may imagine for the non-Aboriginal diggers who discarded the baby rainbow in a rubbish tip. Merlan's account is full of words like "understanding," "viewpoint," "know," "seeing," and "think." This is not surprising given that "the 'inter-' in [her] use of 'intercultural' was modelled after the 'inter-' in intersubjectivity" (169). She assumes that subjectivity "is, of course, 'subject' to the patterning of historical, on-going socio-cultural organization and so not randomly variable" (169). Julie's "affectively and cognitively important understandings of her life" are "generated" in her interactions with Aboriginal and non-Aboriginal people in what may be described as Aboriginal and non-Aboriginal "fields" or settings (e.g., "camp," on the one hand, and "employment," on the other) (171). Patterned subjectivity, which resembles that of others with similar experience in a nonrandom fashion, might be what we call culture, a formulation very similar to those arising from schema theory (e.g., Strauss and Quinn 1994, 1997).[4] Thus we can think of cultural difference, as does Merlan, in terms of divergent experience.

Returning to the idea that we always understand experience in terms of understandings of past experiences (chapter one), it becomes easy to see that although Numbulwar's Aboriginal and non-Aboriginal residents live in an environment that includes practices, arrangements, and institutions such as those of "work," "school," "job," "meeting," "on time," and "debt" as well as "black magic," "ceremony," "curse," "fight," "funeral," and "family," their experiences are shared only to a varying and sometimes quite limited extent. A cultural or intercultural account is premised on the assumption that substantial patterns in this variation will be associated with the identities of "blackfella" and "whitefella."

Merlan (2005) notes that Julie's experiences with "whites" "were mediated by the authority of her old people" (174); so, too, have "the old people" long mediated the experience of Aboriginal people at Numbulwar. Language is perhaps the most obvious example: "Really Kriol is a language. They recognize that Kriol speakers and English speakers often miscommunicate. But I'm not sure if the Numbulwar school teachers got that [from the Kriol workshop]" (DMU 2004). Kriol, the language developed out of the English pidgin spoken by the first children to be schooled at Roper Mission, now Ngurkurr, 155 kilometers southwest of Numbulwar (Harris 1993:149), was the language most commonly spoken in the town during the years of the project. I rarely heard Nunggubuyu spoken by people under the age of forty.

Nunggubuyu, referred to as Wubuy by linguists and increasingly as such by Aboriginal people at Numbulwar,[5] is a prefixing language with multiple noun classes. I know of only one non-Aboriginal person who ever learned to speak it with a degree of fluency—the missionary-linguist, the Reverend Mr. Earl Hughes, who lived and worked at Numbulwar for about seventeen years, producing the first Nunggubuyu-English Dictionary (1971). The following, taken from Heath's (1982) introduction to his Nunggubuyu Dictionary, suggests why this might be the case:

> Nunggubuyu is a language with an extremely large number of phonological rules which often have the effect of altering the surface form of stems in ways which may make it difficult for readers of the texts to identify or reconstruct the correct citation-form representation of the stem and thus find the stem in the dictionary. (xiv)

It has been proposed that the variable bodies of transmissible information we call cultures, and languages as parts of cultures, "tend to become more complex over time." Complexity is constrained, however, by social and cognitive factors, in the latter case by what we may refer to as "cognitive constraints" (Levinson 2006:21–22). In the former case, "contact, trade, and cross-cultural communication" motivate simplification. The development of pidgins as lingua franca provides a prime example of this. The Nunggubuyu language, in contrast, may be an example of cultural complexity that approaches the limit of what the human mind is capable of learning, a complexity that may have arisen from millennia of relative isolation, discussed briefly in the next chapter. It is a language that appears to be nearly impossible for anyone beyond the early years of life to acquire. So it is not surprising that the school has always been taught in English, though from time to time since its start in 1953 (Bayton 1965) there have been special lessons in Wubuy and Aboriginal teaching assistants on hand who might address students in that language. During the years of this study, a bilingual program, known as the "two Way" and understood as a language revitalization effort, was in place and at least some of the teaching assistants used Wubuy, at least some of the time. Most school children, however, along with many of their parents spoke little Wubuy, relying instead on Kriol. All the teaching assistants used Kriol in class. As a part of the bilingual program, the Aboriginal "Numbulwar Community Linguists" included language training in Wubuy for Aboriginal teaching assistants.

I found that some of the women I know who could speak, read, and write English, at least to a limited extent,[6] had children who were not able to do so. Health clinic personnel mentioned that older women routinely accompanied their daughters and grandchildren to serve as translators when they needed medical attention as it was older people who had some English competency, not the younger generations. It seems obvious that a school child or an adult who understands some Wubuy but speaks only Kriol and little or no English likely experiences the school and clinic visits, among other things, in a manner somewhat, if not quite, dissimilar to that of someone who understand only a few words of Wubuy and Kriol, and only speaks English. Similarly, someone who speaks Wubuy and/or Kriol likely understands an Aboriginal ceremony, funeral, or fight in a way that someone who speaks only English does not. This is not an assertion of linguistic relativity or determinism. My point is simply that if you don't understand and speak the language around you, you miss much of what is happening—perhaps, most critically, hints of just what actions and events mean to people who are speaking in a language you don't understand.

Whitefella Things

[Young people] are going to start taking off and travelling and they are gonna have trouble because the culture here is so communal, looking after [them] and they get jealous if anybody gets too much. It's so competitive in the city. Life is so much more competitive and if they end up in cities, even after [school] here they are going to have to be more competitive and work harder. People freak out when I tell them how much it costs for a house. You have to save $50,000 for a down payment and [pay the mortgage] every month. It seems too hard, so they'll just live here. And they have to learn the value of money . . . If they want cars, furniture, they have to learn a work ethic and city competitiveness. The whole thing is cultural. They are so lucky to have strong family, beautiful bush, beautiful country, but everything is changing so quickly. (UTG 2005)

Numbulwar is not "the city," but most of its infrastructure has been created and maintained by outsiders who have always been non-Indigenous in outlook, and sometimes unsympathetic to an Aboriginal perspective, according to rules and routines that remain foreign to many, if not most, of the Aboriginal people I know.

As a physical entity, Numbulwar is very much a whitefella creation of public buildings, houses, and roads. These are scattered across not quite two square kilometers of sand dunes on the western shore of the Gulf of Carpentaria. The original "Village," housing Aboriginal people in the 1950s, had by 2003 expanded to become the four housing areas of "Bottom Camp," "Top Camp," "Middle Camp," and "New Town." Aboriginal people had resided in the once exclusively whitefella occupied "Missionarea" from the 1980s onward. By the late 1990s, whitefellas lived in houses among those occupied by Aboriginal people in New Town and Middle Camp. What may be regarded as the town center is defined by buildings and associated institutions of whitefella society: the school, the clinic, the Council office complex, the police station, and the shop.

Covering an area approximately the size of a large city block, the buildings of Numbulwar's school have always, to my Western eyes, presented a picture of wealth and well-being, a picture in startling contrast to the relative disorder, dirt, and material poverty of most of Numbulwar's homes. Its buildings are substantial, its floors and walls relatively clean, its grounds relatively clear of litter. The classrooms are well lighted and air-conditioned, the furnishings colorful. Educational items—paper, pens, pencils, paints, musical instruments, and books among other things—have always seemed in plentiful supply. We might interpret the school's relative splendor and its central location as a sign of the importance that whitefellas have long placed on the education of Aboriginal people. Certainly, the missionaries who established Rose River Mission saw Western education as central to their effort: "The native people still live in their own way, but with the constant teaching, especially of the children, we naturally expect results in due course" (Montgomerie, Annual Report 1954, in Cole 1982:34). Staffed, as has long been the case, by teachers from the Northern Territory Department of Education, the school had classes for children from the age of three, who might attend "Infants," often accompanied by their mothers, through to young adults, age eighteen and over, who attended the "Post Primary" classes, along with younger teens. The post primary program included a "Corro," or "Correspondence Course," for the half dozen or so students regarded by the teaching staff as particularly promising.

Ever since I have been visiting Numbulwar, the school's teachers have spoken of attendance as a problem. In 2003, I was told that the number of children coming to school was between 120 and 130, though a larger number was enrolled and at one point in the previous year, attendance had fallen to as low as 50 or 60. Children might be taken out of school when their parents traveled, either to another, usually nearby, community or outstation. A whole classroom might be almost, if not entirely, empty for days because girls in the class had been fighting. When a *Kunabibi* ceremony was held in 2005 at a homeland about fifty kilometers away, school attendance was affected by the exodus of men, women, and school-aged children. In 1978, the school principal would walk or drive through the Village ringing a bell, calling out that children were not coming to school and should do so. In the years of this study, teachers attempted to attract children with a music program, outings, and prizes for coming to school. Such methods were not always effective however. "And the boys. They know they are off to Garma [Festival] and really looking forward to it and the day before they are to go, the ganja comes to town. Three boys went and got stoned and didn't come to school the day they were flying out to Garma" (ITU 2003). In the post primary grade, at least some of the teachers said that the separation of boys and girls had led to better attendance. No longer were the girls such easy targets of the boys" "punches," and the gender segregation made it easier to make classes "more interesting" for both boys and girls. Girls, it was said, did not, for example, display the same enthusiasm that boys did for the music classes taught by two local young men. Still, at least one teacher wondered about her students. "Sometimes I don't know why they come to school. Must be nothing else to do...They are in such a strange place. They've had TV, DVD, CD, mobile phones and it's all happened so fast. They don't know where to take direction from" (ITU 2004). She also wondered about the school's effects, if not intentions:

> We're trying to educate students to a high level and what this does is raise the level of frustration and here there is no pathway, no jobs, no one to hire our students. The community doesn't have a mine, a source of money, there is nothing here. No infrastructure. I don't see where the education is leading. These kids put all this effort into education and end up on CDP [i.e., CDEP, Community Development Employment Projects] collecting trash. (ITU 2003)[7]

Also located in the center of town are the Council offices and the shop. The Council is comprised of people from "clans" associated with the land where Numbulwar is located and the countryside around it.[8] At least in theory, it replaced the governing power of the Mission superintendent, a change that took place in the late 1970s (Burbank 1988). Notable in the years of this study was not simply the number of women on this body, which at most of the meetings I attended was a majority, but the fact that they were a part of what had once been a completely male institution.

At the Council's front office, people could pick up the mail (flown into town, usually three times a week), buy stamps, access the cash machine, and, if they were lucky, use the office phone or fax.[9] The air-conditioned building also contained the Town Clerk's office, an office occupied by the Community Development Employment Projects (CDEP) manager, one by several Indigenous and non-Indigenous office workers who, among other things, worked on Council accounts, and one for the Numbulwar Council President, who has always been an Aboriginal man elected by Numbulwar's Aboriginal population. There was a toilet and a meeting room that ran along the back of the building, its veranda overlooking the sea and the oldest part of town. A loudspeaker was kept in the Council office. It was used by the Council president or another community member to broadcast news or comment. It was from this loudspeaker that people might learn that there was a "body comin," that a corpse was arriving, most likely from the Darwin hospital, for burial in the community.

The shop was located across the road from the Council office. With its wide sheltered terrace on two sides, tables and benches and the "fast food" window—where people could buy soft drinks, cigarettes, hamburgers, barbequed chicken, and the like—the shop was a good place to find people, especially during school recess. School children and adults seemed to prefer the fast food to the relatively low-fat snacks available in the school's "tuck shop," if the numbers standing in their respective lines were any indication. Groups of senior men would gather on the shop's veranda, as would groups of women, family clusters, children, and dogs.

Saturday, October 29, 2005

[At shop] my bill is a shock, $58. I ask for price of packet of chicken wings—about 6 wings—told $6. Turns out oysters i.e. tin of smoked oysters are $5 each. I've got 4 tins. A glance at shelf suggested they were $1.85/tin. Price of head of lettuce is $4.50. (2005:1:23)

As this journal entry suggests, prices in the Numbulwar shop were somewhat higher than they would have been in a major Australian city at the time. At least some Aboriginal people thought so as well.

> *Sherry*: That shop in Numbulwar, here, is too dear. Because if you wanna buy maybe TV or video maybe it cost you a lot of money.
> *Kinsey*: And you come back la [from the] shop, no change. (Sherry and Kinsey 2005)

The fortnightly barge from Darwin carried the individual shopping orders (mostly whitefella's) along with those of the community's shop and various workshops. I always found it an impressive sight; its red painted bulk sometimes remained in view for hours as it waited for a tidal change in the Gulf that would allow it to enter the Rose River mouth, dock, and unload at the "jetty." Occasionally, supplies reached Numbulwar overland from Darwin or Katherine via the road intersecting the Stuart Highway near Mataranka, which leads first to Ngukurr and then to Numbulwar. Not surprisingly, transportation to Numbulwar is costly. The shop, owned by the Numbulwar Council and run by whitefella managers, included the cost of transportation in its pricing.[10]

During the years of this study, the shop stocked a greater supply and variety of foods than I had seen on my earlier visits. The freezers contained cuts of beef, chicken, and lamb as well as sausage and mince, vegetables, ice cream, and cakes. Loaves of bread, butter, margarine, cheese, eggs, nuts, dried fruit, breakfast cereal, long-life if not fresh milk, both whole and skim, were usually available, as were a variety of fresh, if somewhat wilted, fruits and vegetables, a state in which they arrived, to judge from the quality of similar items I received directly from the barge. The Coke, other soft drinks, and dry goods I remembered from before—the barrels of flour, bags of sugar and rice, cartons of tea leaves, and tins of instant coffee—were usually in plentiful supply.[11]

Items of Western material culture have, from its inception as Rose River Mission, been present at Numbulwar and, as will be seen in following chapters, have long had practical and emotional significance in people's lives. During the study years, many if not most people owned or had access to vehicles, televisions, video players, DVDs, CD or tape players, washing machines, and electric stoves. The shop stocked such goods as refrigerators, clothing and shoes, bed frames, blankets, brooms, pots and pans, cooking implements, cups and plates, flatware, children's toys, and the plastic flowers people used to decorate the church for funerals, and to place on the "coffin box" at the point in the service that was referred to as "flower time." When checks arrived in the mail or were available for access at the "TCU", the Traditional Credit Union, the shop would fill, mostly with women, pushing carts filled with groceries.

When I arrived for the last fieldwork period of the study in 2005, work had stopped on a police station that was being built on the empty concrete foundation of the old shop next door to the Council office. The construction workers, I was told, were "on strike" to protest the recurrent destruction, presumably wrought by local youths, which routinely undid what they had done. One woman joked that she would be the first to stay in the police station. Another, however, told me that people were "gonna run away," "they are frightened," "they don't like to stay," because "they are building police station."

People didn't run away and by the time of my visit in 2007, two young men had qualified as police aides to assist the two regular police officers who rotated through the community from relatively nearby places—Katherine, Mataranka, Groote Island, and Ngukurr—for a month at a time. Numbulwar has long had Aboriginal police aides (usually local men) in residence, though not on a continuous basis. The two new regular police officers, however, were the first to reside full time, round the clock. In previous years, Aboriginal people were, in line with their status as state wards, under Mission authority backed by visiting "welfare" officers and police (Burbank 1988, 1994). In later years, authority rested with the Aboriginal Council, a council that has always been headed or assisted by a whitefella, either as superintendent or as town clerk. When serious crimes such as assault and murder were committed, police on Groote Eylandt or at Ngukurr were called. They might arrive, of course, many hours, if not days, later.

In chapter four, I detail the extent to which cannabis use is perceived as a problem by many people at Numbulwar. During my brief visit in 2007, women told me, with what seemed like relief, that people, their close kin included, were no longer smoking it. "Ganja mob *gotnot* ganja cause of the police, so they fishing now and playing card now. If they wanna smoke [cannabis] they go to Groote and Ngukurr" (2007:II:53). The police were checking vehicles and the bags of people traveling in by air, confiscating not only drugs and alcohol, a prohibited substance in this "dry" community,[12] but also the vehicles used to import them. The actions of the sniffer dog used both at the Groote Island and Numbulwar airstrips were explained to me: "When the plane landed they lined up all the bags and the dog was happy for that bag, he sat down and barked" (2007:II:57). In the yard used to store impounded vehicles behind the police station, I counted two cars, two trucks, and one dinghy.

People were not always happy with police practice, however. A meeting helped the police understand that "old men" have sacred "thing" stored in their houses and the police were acting "too hard" when they searched houses for alcohol and drugs. A woman protested about the way they dealt with her son when he was drawn into what sounded like a drunken brawl. At another meeting, men were said to be "angry," and "old ladies" "growling" because the police had checked the bags their sons brought with them when they returned from Borroloola; their sons, they said, had gone to a funeral, and "don't smoke ganja."

Some months later, telephone conversations informed me that cannabis was back in town and indicated its use was as widespread as before. Perhaps the dry season roads provided greater opportunity for bringing it into the community again, as both blackfellas and whitefellas had predicted they would. Or perhaps the police cohort in charge at the time was not as dedicated to, or practiced at, preventing its distribution in the town.

Not only are the physical structures of Numbulwar whitefella creations, many of its practices largely derive from Western social arrangements. For example, the primary subsistence source for most Aboriginal people has long been various forms of welfare. Merry and Sherry, close kin and good friends—women I have known since they were small children—often spoke of "Pension Week" and "UB [unemployment benefits] Week," pointing out the "P" and "V/F" on alternating weeks of the calendars I always brought with me, symbols I had not noticed before. Pension and unemployment money was referred to as "pay," as in "I got my pay today." However, Kinsey, a younger woman, distinguished between money received for working, referred to as "sweating money," and money simply received: "When you working, that's sweating, comes from your body. That sweating money, from working, not royalty money" (2007 I:4–5). Some people at Numbulwar did earn sweating money. In 2003 there were about seventy workers on CDEP, thirty women and forty men, doing twenty different kinds of work around the community. These jobs included managing Centrelink (the social security and services office), grading roads, fencing, landscaping yards and public spaces, carpentry, welding, and working in the clinic as health workers. By "royalty money," Kinsey refers to the money that some people, those with kinship connections to Groote or Bickerton islands, received from GEMCO (the Groote Eylandt Mining Company), a manganese mining enterprise on Groote Eylandt, about sixty-five kilometers offshore.[13]

A Sustainable Way of Life?

One day I asked a senior Aboriginal man of my acquaintance the following question: "What do you think would happen to Numbulwar if the government stopped all the money for the Council, CDP, the school, the hospital [clinic]; if people here only had money from UB, child welfare and pension money?" He replied as follows:

> SM: I guess we would look elsewhere for assistance, we would look to some of the big banks. They are offering, two banks in Australia, has offered assistance in providing assistance to any community...Once you get the money, they will assist you too with funding whichever way you want to use it...Once you are up and running, then they will leave you on your own.
> VKB: If you got assistance from the bank, what would you create with the money?
> SM: We have potential like crayfish, farming crayfish, we can breed barramundi or crabs, tourism and all these other big businesses in the Territory. We can start up international markets, create international markets like bush medicine. All of these things we have in our resources. Plus minerals. We have gold, bauxite, manganese, we have that here...We do have a lot of options. If government departments will change about money, we have a lot of other options. We have resources here. There are a lot of resources. We can go to a bank or a mining company and have a partnership, so there are a lot of options if it come to that stage. We need to put this up in our vision statement. We need to talk about it now. If Council decide we don't need any more handouts from government departments, now is the time for everybody to start thinking about education, training, apprenticeships, work toward achieving. (SM2004)

Among other things, this man's reply to my question reiterates the teacher's statement: Numbulwar neither has nor provides its population with a sustainable material base. Its existence, much like Darwin's—the capital city of the Northern Territory—is the result of bureaucratic fiat, just as the material existence of its population, whitefellas and blackfellas alike, derives largely, if not exclusively, from one form of Territory or Commonwealth funding or another. Of greatest interest, however, is his vision of a future that is cast neither in terms of a return to past activities of hunting and gathering nor in a move to "the city." In casting the future of its Aboriginal population in situ, it reflects the views of people I know, and, I suspect, most of Numbulwar's other Aboriginal residents, though the whitefella anticipating young people's moves to "the city" might disagree. For example, I asked eight women if they would "like to move to Darwin, Katherine, Gove or some other town to live." All replied in the negative.[14] Staying at Numbulwar, however, requires more than a foraging based economy. In pre-mission times, groups of several hundred people were able to remain in the area where the town is now situated for several months at certain times of year, indicating that, at least in some seasons, this Arnhem Land environment provided an abundance not always found in hunting and gathering settings (Biernoff 1979:156). Nevertheless, it seems highly improbable that an exclusive pursuit of hunting and gathering activities could adequately provide for a population of 800, often augmented by up to around 200 visitors.[15] The people at Numbulwar and its associated outstations who continue to hunt and gather do not sustain themselves with these activities.

For the most part, the Aboriginal people of Numbulwar are also not engaged in the "real economy" (Pearson 2000). They are, however, very much engaged in "consumer society." Some of this consumption arises simply from a need for such basics as food and shelter in circumstances where past economic practices are no longer viable. But another form of consumption is apparent at Numbulwar as well. Kawachi and Kennedy (2002) argue that intense competition for "positional goods," things "we value because others do not have them" (70), is particularly likely to arise in circumstances of inequality. Thinking of the egalitarian ethos that generally characterizes Aboriginal communities, of the pressures to share and emotions such as "shame" and "jealous" associated with attempts to address perceived imbalance, we might first question the relevance of this argument for Numbulwar. Kawachi and Kennedy themselves would seem to exclude people somewhat like remote community Aboriginal people when they use the following statement from Sen (1992):

> While the rural Indian may have little problem in appearing in public without shame with relatively modest clothing and can take part in the life of the community without a telephone or a television, the

commodity requirements of these general functionings are much more demanding in a country where people standardly use a bigger basket of diverse commodities (In Kawachi and Kennedy 2003:65)

We must keep in mind, however, not simply the relatively egalitarian sociality of Aboriginal people but also the presence of whitefellas and a history and significance of whitefella culture in blackfella lives. It is hard to imagine that the material abundance of Western culture, whether this consists of multiple room dwellings, well-functioning vehicles, or sophisticated communication equipment, is not noted by people who so recently relied on hunting and gathering, an economic strategy generally associated with a practical and sparse material culture. When such material abundance is coupled with the status and power differentials of blackfellas/whitefellas, though some facets of these may today be more imagined than real, it is not surprising that many whitefella things become the object of blackfella desires: "Girls ask for some things they've seen on TV, always beauty items, face creams for example. Usually I can't get them. They are specialized items. Usually its girls wanting things they've seen" (STL 2005). Richerson and Boyd (2005), along with generations of advertising executives, have observed what may be a pan-human potential, if not propensity, to "imitate the successful" (125). We can see these girls attempting, though without success, to imitate the behavior of high prestige people, models on TV. From the perspective of evolutionary theory, however, the utility of such a strategy depends on a positive "correlation between the traits that *indicate* success and the traits that *cause* success." When this is not the case, "prestige bias" "can lead to an unstable, runaway process" (124–5).

Whether or not consumer society is "an unstable, runaway process," most Aboriginal people at Numbulwar are ill prepared to engage in this form of competition because their access to the means of doing so—money—is limited. Only the relatively few on CDEP and employed at the school may receive amounts above those received from the various forms of welfare. Generally, levels of educational achievement and English competency make employment outside the community a rare possibility, assuming a willingness, rarely apparent, to leave Numbulwar or cognate communities for prolonged periods of time. Those who receive royalties do so rarely, and the egalitarian ethos of the family network usually ensures that substantial sums soon diffuse. The limited funds provided by welfare are all that most of Numbulwar's potential consumers have to look forward to in the present and foreseeable future.[16]

Funerals

Funerals, occurring throughout the study period with what seems like disturbing regularity, provided an intercultural setting for the social and the sacred, moments in community life when the juxtaposition of at least two belief systems could be seen: the Indigenous belief system, referred to at Numbulwar as "Law," and the form of Christianity introduced originally by the Anglican missionaries, modified over the years by both blackfella and whitefella congregants. There were, of course, variations in each funeral that I attended,[17] but there were coexisting, if not intersecting, patterns in them as well, what might be thought of as the Christian pattern and the Law or Culture pattern.[18]

> From 12:00 on I listen for church bells, go out on veranda to see if anything happening around church. Around 2:00 I hear prayer coming from church. As I'm just putting on [funeral] clothes, hear [kin term directed at me] at front door. Grab things, go out…they've come for me for the funeral. Brady, [Teejay's younger sister, about age twelve] and [her younger male cousin]. Ask where Brady's mother sitting. Brady responds that [her mother's sister and sister-in-law] are in church, though [one of these women] said sitting in the church makes them "too sad." Brady tells me, "It's a white box. They talk talk, then flower time." We go behind church, various groups sitting out on sand. I see [a whitefella] in one group. Can't spot Brady's mother. Brady says under the tamarind tree. (2005 II:77)

People might choose to sit either in or outside the church during a funeral; many, especially men, children, and adolescents, would spend some time inside and some time out. Outside one was more able to see and hear the procession of men who had collected the body from the mortuary just across a sand hill from the church hall, placed it in a vehicle and accompanied it, singing the public clan songs[19] of the deceased en route to the church. Outside might also be a place where people, like a deceased man's sisters and wives, once expected to stay away from a "brother's" or "husband's" funeral, might sit. It was also a place where people apparently felt more able to smoke, eat and drink, and talk than they did inside the church building.

Younger men acted as pallbearers, generally entering the church only long enough to place the coffin on a table, covered with a white cloth, in the center aisle. Their entrance was greeted by the local or visiting Aboriginal priest and the wails of the principal mourners, "close family," who might put their arms around each other as they cried. People might also embrace the coffin resting their head upon it once it was set down. The older men who had accompanied the coffin to the church would retire to the shade of a nearby house or tree. The songs they continued to sing, along with the accompanying sound of clap sticks, could be heard intermittently throughout the service, whether one was sitting inside or out.

Inside the church, the service proceeded much as my young companion Brady said it did: "talk talk then flower time." The Aboriginal priests, whether local or from neighboring communities, used their funeral orations to rebuke gamblers and ganja smokers or entreat people to turn away from the Law and to Christianity.

> After you die, God decides where you are going to go, what country you are going to stay in. If you go down into everlasting eternal fire, down and down maybe you are going to call out to Jesus then to save you. But he will say "No!" I look at you and I see pretty face, pretty outside, but ugly inside. I can't see inside. But you have to have God inside, not just to speak. (2003 V:21)

> The Lord is coming back, coming back to this country. We don't know when. We have to be ready. If we are ready, we can't die. It doesn't matter if we jump in the river, hang ourself, cut ourself, we will live. If we aren't ready, like most people here, we will go to hell. We have to get ready by believing in him. It can't be your mother, it can't be your father, it can't be your family. You have to do it yourself. It can't come from them, it has to come from you. (2004 IX:34)[20]

The priests or officiating deacons invited others to talk, and some did, though far more briefly than the priests. Like the priest, they usually addressed the coffin by the kin term with which they had once addressed the deceased, and sometimes explained their kin connection at some length. People were also called upon to provide music, and always did. Bands supplied with electric guitars, keyboards, and amplifiers played either Christian or popular pieces, often, if not exclusively, of local composition, and women, well practiced from frequent evening Fellowship meetings, always provided Christian songs and hymns via handheld microphones.

There is a River, known as the "flower song," signaled "flower time." People, generally family, walked into the center of the church and placed plastic flowers upon the coffin, sometimes wailing and falling upon it. The flowers were soon removed to be placed in the waiting vehicle, as was the coffin, again taken up by the pallbearers who reentered the church to do so. Wailing and embracing the coffin occurred throughout this phase of the ritual. This was also the time when on two occasions I observed male kin of the deceased gesturing with weapons and haranguing the crowd about their neglect and abuse of the men being buried that day. One of these deceased had died as a result of being stabbed while he was in Darwin; the other had been embroiled, several years before his death, in a community-wide dispute over Numbulwar's ownership. These gestures were expected, physical expressions of being "sorry an' wild," emotions that I have often seen and heard articulated at the time of a man's death at Numbulwar. The fearsome and ritual nature of such a display by one of these men, who gestured with a sword and a knife, was both undermined and underlined by the placid infant he held in his arms at the same time.

The church and its surrounds would empty as people followed the de facto hearse making its way slowly down Wandarang Road toward the cemetery, perhaps a half kilometer away from the southern edge of town. Wandarang Road would be edged with small piles of dried grass and moiety-specific leaves and, as the vehicle moved along, these piles were ignited by men who had originally brought the coffin from the mortuary to the church. This group continued singing as they walked, stopping occasionally to dance an accompaniment to their songs. The road by this time would be lined with people who had not come to the church service but might at this point join in the procession and the dancing.

At the town's southern limits, the funeral cortege would stop. Several songs would be played and dances danced. For one man, his "mother song," that is, a clan song of his long deceased mother, was performed; "his mother saying good bye to him." The "spear Dance" was performed to the "*Wungarri* [fight/anger] Song" played at several funerals because the "old man" who had died was a "warrior." At this juncture in the procession, I saw older people being helped into the vehicle for a minute or two, as though to give them one last chance to see the coffin and be with the deceased. Men and women might again express their distress and anger for the death of a family member loudly and dramatically, with gestures that sometimes mimicked acts of physical aggression. Following the final acts consisting of growls and shouts, "pushing the body, it's ready to go," the hearse continued toward the cemetery, now accompanied by only those people who regard themselves one way or another as "right" or "close" family of the dead. In the cemetery, the coffin was lowered into the grave, excavated from whatever sand hill it was located on by a backhoe, and buried to the accompaniment of an Anglican service conducted by the officiating priest. People who attended this part of the funeral might, following this service, visit the graves of family members, identified occasionally by wooden crosses with names carved upon them, or more simply by the location of sun faded plastic flower arrangements on the sand.

Change

Funerals as intercultural sites enable us to see something of the complexity and complications of cultural processes that inexorably lead to changes in Aboriginal lives (see Macdonald 2001:182, 188).

The rhythm of daily life in the town, at least during daylight hours, is to a great extent a whitefella creation and probably always has been. Once, the Council building, located in the same place as the current one but then an older structure, was fronted by a tower bearing a siren. On my first trip to Numbulwar in 1977, the siren sounded five times a day, except on weekends when only the church bell rang; then the siren was audible to all as Numbulwar covered much less ground, consisting only of the 'Missionarea" and "Aboriginal housing." The first siren, at 7:45 a.m., signaled that work and school would soon begin. The last, at 5:00 p.m., informed people that the community's shop was now closed. In the study period the shop still closed at 5:00 on weekdays, but there was no longer a siren to signal this. Perhaps because the siren had disappeared some years ago, the school played a recording of a bell, later one of piano music, to indicate that school was beginning or resuming after the morning break. When, however, a "body" came to town, as one did on seven occasions during the seven months of fieldwork for this study, the predominantly whitefella routines of Numbulwar ceased, at least for a while.

Sounds permeated the thin fibro walls and tin roof of the small Health Department flat that I was able to use during my stays in town and flowed through the gaps of the louvered windows even when they were closed during cooler weather. The most consistent of these were of people: talking, laughing, yelling, and fighting. Dogs often barked, and music played, sometimes for hours on end, usually from a neighbor's stereo or CD player. On some nights the sound of music, particularly the base notes, came from "New Town" when the Yilila band performed or from the disco at the Recreation Hall near the shop; sometimes it came from the portable CD players adolescents carried with them in their nocturnal meetings on the sand hills behind the flat.[21] In 2007 it came from a vehicle or two equipped with stereos.

On Sunday mornings I knew when church service was about to begin, both from the bell that gave warning that the time was near and from the procession of Christians who walked down the road: the wives of MAF (Mission Aviation Fellowship) pilots with their children, other whitefellas, an Aboriginal man or maybe two, at least twice as many Aboriginal women, and a handful of Aboriginal children on their way to Sunday school. If I stood at the end of the open back veranda of the flat, I could see the "church hall" and church itself, large wooden and fibro buildings, simple and shed-like, both in shape and in the use of corrugated iron roofs. When funerals were held, I could tell from the sounds of the bell and the amplified music that always accompanied them that it was time for me to go to the church for one of the six I was expected to attend during the course of the study.

Most of the sounds I could hear in the flat diminished or disappeared completely when a body, refrigerated in the mortuary, located next to the clinic and referred to as the "moke house," was awaiting burial. At such a time, people were to show "respect" to the deceased and to the family of the deceased; they should not "laugh or make noise." Not everyone conformed to this rule, however. I frequently heard people talking and laughing during the period when a body was awaiting burial. In one case, my neighbor maintained his music's volume over several days, though there was a body in the mortuary almost next door. In another, the grandchildren responsible for making the necessary funeral arrangements for the deceased, a man of considerable ritual status, rebuked townspeople on the Council's loudspeaker and threatened to throw spears if their noisy and disrespectful behavior continued.

Once, in such circumstances, all public buildings at Numbulwar would have been closed until the funeral was held; once people would have stayed close to home, if not actually inside. The shop would not sell food or tobacco, the school would not open its doors, nor would the clinic and the Council offices. Tap water could not be used, nor could people walk in certain places until smoking rituals were performed to remove the sacred and dangerous aspects brought to these locales by death. During the years of this study, however, only during a "day of respect" and during the time of the funeral itself were the school, clinic, office, and shop closed. The shop, for example, might be opened in the morning, though a funeral was scheduled for the afternoon, if, say, people had received their "pay" that day. Discos, concerts, or birthday parties might be held on the same day as a funeral once its rites were completed.

Women regarded as widows were still expected to "hide," though no longer covered with the clay needed to prevent the deceased from returning to them (a practice of which I've only been told). Nor were women expected to withdraw in the discomfort of the bush, but, rather, in their own homes unless it was also that of the deceased. The house of a dead man was rarely the home of all of his wives. Many widows are classificatory "wives" ('sisters," most often, of a man's actual wife), women who once could have been co-wives in a polygynous union. These, however, were extremely rare during the study years, with only one or two men identified as having more than one wife.

On one occasion, a woman married to a classificatory brother of the deceased chose not to hide, attending a course she was taking in Darwin instead. She may not, however, have done this with impunity; it was rumored that her husband gave her a beating upon her return. Similarly, people might not return to Numbulwar for funerals if they were otherwise occupied in town; sometimes they would call to say they were "sorry" they could not come. "No money" for travel was a reason that might be given and accepted, at least in theory, without offense. In past years, I had seen a house or two in considerable disrepair bulldozed after a death, but during the time of this study, houses were not destroyed, though they would be vacated for a period of time. At a later date, after being "smoked" they could be reinhabited, though not usually by "close" kin of the deceased who would still be feeling "too sad" and "sorry."

Clearly some of these changes have been made in response to the requirements of whitefella ways and the constraints these have introduced in blackfella lives. The shorter length of time that the shop remained closed probably indicates the extent to which people had come to rely on it for food and other basic items. Other changes, particularly what might be described as the disrespectful behavior of the young, might instead be described as "culture loss," as indeed they are by some Aboriginal people.

It has now been many years since Keen (in Hiatt 1985:43–4), Myers (1980:211–12), and Sackett (1978:116) suggested that the efficacy of initiation into a male ritual hierarchy as a means of social control relies on the Law's exclusive hold on the minds of initiates. The introduction of multiple discourses enables an agency that may not always be to the benefit of a community.

There are reasons why our young kids have gone on their own path. They broke away from our culture, they can do anything. That makes

me wonder why they doing that. They can go and sniff petrol anytime they want, to smoke ganja anytime they want to. If they feel like
smoking ganja, we can't stop them; they can drink alcohol anytime
they want. They can play music of the tape recorder, big stereo they
can buy from the shop. They can play music loud as they like it any
time. They don't worry about the next door neighbour. They can
choose whatever woman they want to meet during the day or the
night. And all these other things that young people does that I see
them do, it's completely out of my reach. I can't hold them up and say
to them, "You should be doing that." Us mob today, we don't have
any power to do anything. Our power system was lost as soon as we
lost the elders to control the community. (Sawyer 2003)

Other changes, however, might be seen, in a more positive light,
as cultural innovation. Once, by custom, certain people—"sisters"
and "wives" and children—were excluded from funerals. During the
study years, however, "You see now, see biggest mob of women and
children all there. Young people too, they weren't allowed [before]
unless they were chosen by the person who looks after the ceremony of the dead person" (Sawyer 2004). We might view the current
form taken by funerals, specifically the inclusion of a greater range
of people in their ritual, as an indication of the continuing, if not
increasing, importance of family, a theme I shall return to again and
again in this book.[22] In this context, it is worth taking a closer look
at the word "respect."

> *VKB*: What happens if you should do something [for funeral prepara-
> tions] and you don't?
> *Merry*: Maybe if you won't do it, if, family, will get upset. Maybe
> growl at you and they say, "Why didn't you respect, he's your own
> uncle, gagu [kin term]," like that. Every time people died, you
> gotta respect, all the time.
> *VKB*: How do you say "respect" in Nunggubuyu?
> *Merry*: Babumamani, you help them. You mob gotta help them. If
> you respect them and help them, they won't be upset. You showing
> respect to them. So family gonna be happy and realize. Maybe peo-
> ple get worried if someone doesn't help, "Why the man won't help
> us, he's related to him, he should be respect!" "You didn't help us
> yesterday," they say, "because you didn't respect us." (Merry 2005)

Respect is a word that appears to have only recently entered the
vocabulary of people at Numbulwar, at least in relation to their
mortuary practices. Few of the people I asked to translate it into
Wubuy or Kriol could, and the translations I did receive varied.

Heath (1982) does not include it in his English-to-Nunggubuyu dictionary. In Merry's usage of it, respect for the dead is simultaneously respect for surviving family. It is manifest as "help" that makes family of the dead "happy," assisting the dead to separate from the living, and vice versa.

For several days prior to the funeral service, clan songs and dances are staged around the residence of the deceased; soon before it, *arnag* is performed: "The corroboree goes on for maybe three or four days. Then when the main part comes, they gotta, if the dead person touched them, a lot of people have smoking ceremony so the dead person can't see them. They callem *arnag*" (Sawyer 2004). Originally, *arnag* for widows was delayed long past the burial, but in recent times widows are painted and cleansed with smoke before the funeral rites: "They do *arnag* before the body goes to cemetery, because *ngayi* [widow] want to see the body too, that's why they sing the *wunubal* [public clan songs (Heath 1982:269)] to *ngayi* mob, to paint them red one [with ochre], so they can see it" (Sherry and Merry 2005). Sawyer, a man in his fifties, describes himself as a "leader" of his clan. Here is his explanation for this change:

> This widow never used to come out when they take the box to the burial place. That happens after when they have a corroboree to release the *ngayi*. Because *ngayi* is most important people. The widow has been with him from the start. So we have to change the rule. So now she has to be there to see the body, but not to stand too close. (Sawyer 2004) (cf. Barber 2008:162)

Musing on the extent to which Martu people in Western Australia dedicate significant and scarce resources to the mortuary practices that are taking place within an epidemic of premature mortality similar to that experienced at Numbulwar, M. Tonkinson (2008) says, "It is as if they have chosen to deal with a reality they feel helpless to alter by applying their energy and skills to making it a celebration of who they are" (52). The same might be said of the people at Numbulwar, and who they are is predominantly family. Others writing on the subject of mortuary practices in Indigenous Australia have made similar points (see Glaskin et al. 2008). Useful here is the connection that Macdonald (2008) draws between attendance at Wiradjuri funerals and "demand sharing" (discussed further in chapter four). This conceptual equation helps us see that respect is an act of a kind with those that create, maintain, and symbolize the importance of Aboriginal relationships to Aboriginal people, acts of particular importance at a time when family is assailed by death (see Bowlby 1980; Malinowski 1948).

At the same time, we might note the introjection of what has been identified in some forms of Christianity as the "value of individualism" (Robbins 2007:307) in one of a priest's funeral exhortations: "We have to get ready by believing in him. It can't be your mother, it can't be your father, it can't be your family. You have to do it yourself. It can't come from them, it has to come from you" (2004:IX:34). While some view Christianity as an antidote to the antisocial behavior displayed by some of the young,[23] the individualism of its message could be made instead to support precisely those kinds of actions.

The intercultural domain is clearly a complicated one, not least because there is not a consensus about changes that might be introduced. Here, for example, Majiwi, a woman in her fifties, speaks about a meeting that she and other "Christian women" held with an Aboriginal priest.

> Reverend been [holding a] meeting for *wunubal* to stop. Church can take over [funeral matters]. "We can't give you the answer," we said, and, "talk to the men." They might blame the Christian women. They've been putting the pressure on us. Don't know what the story gonna be. Numbulwar got most, got culture. Groote and Umbakumba really forgetting [culture] now.[24] Groote they are using people from Numbulwar [to dance and sing] for funerals. We understand Christian life. God has given us those culture things. Those Jews people. They keep their laws. I told [that] old man, "this is wrong and you making it hard for *wuruwuruj* [blackfellas] to stop that culture stuff." Long time ago, man passed away, widow had to go out. To clean up and put the string [*jirward*, a string collar worn by widows] and paint up. That's always passed on. No one can stop that one. (Majiwi 2004)

One of the Anglican priests serving at Numbulwar held a meeting with church women to discuss the matter of mortuary and mourning practices. It appears that the vestment of widows with a string collar of multiple strands and red ochre was among the forms that he suggested should be abandoned. Majiwi did not agree with this, and argued that people can maintain their culture and be Christian at the same time. After all, she argued, "God has given us those culture things" and no one should stop these practices. In any event, the women didn't want to be blamed for making the decision, and told the "Reverend" to "talk to the men."

The intercultural domain is also a complicated one because the sources of change do not necessarily match up with blackfella and whitefella identities. The argument about acceptable funeral practices, which clearly originates in whitefella culture, was promoted by an Anglican priest who would be identified by many, himself included, as a blackfella.

Blackfella Values, Whitefella Things

Speaking, for the most part, with reference to policy papers and other forms of "officialese," Sutton (2009) says that:

> [Causal theories of] Indigenous disadvantage, especially in the field of Indigenous health...[have] rested on a cultural flat earth, one in which the particular values and types of social organization of the colonized and of the colonizers were of no importance in understating why different populations reacted to being overrun by different conquering people in such markedly different ways. (81)

The idea of "values," generally accompanied by an assumption that those arising from different sociocultural formations may when juxtaposed be "incompatible" or "in conflict," has long been used as a conceptual tool in anthropological analyses of social and cultural changes. For example, in a study resting upon a premise derived from Kluckhohn and Strodtbeck (1961) that values are "rank ordered" (4), Hausfeld (1977:287) looked for and found significant correlations between "value dissonance" and ill health (used as an indicator of stress) for groups of Aboriginal and non-Aboriginal Australians. His conclusion that "stress does not result from change but rather from its absence when the environment demands it" foreshadows the argument that I shall present in chapters six and seven. Similarly in concert with this line of thought, Austin Broos (2009) sees the "radical marginalization" of Arrente people as a consequence of being "encompassed entirely in a cash economy...because the forms of value they brought from the past could no longer redefine their circumstances"; they remain, at least in part, embedded in "relatedness and their emplaced identities within a local region" (5, 7).

"Take [Aboriginal woman]. Yesterday, someone bugged her for money, she just took off [from her job]. We've said to them, 'Just let us know when you are going. Maybe we can help you.' They have lots of family problems" (STL 2005). Though at least some blackfellas worked and earned money, and all purchased and used items of Western material culture, it cannot be assumed that work and money and Western things mean more or less the same things to both white-fellas and blackfellas at Numbulwar. There are many reasons why this might be so. Whitefellas are more likely to hold positions of relative power and authority than local people. They are more likely than locals to have received substantial training and recognition for the work they do. They usually earn more money, and are likely to have fewer demands placed upon the money they make and the things they already own or buy than their Aboriginal coworkers. Beyond these contrasts in blackfella and whitefella circumstances, however, may lie not so much different values as distinct hierarchies of value.

A sentence in which Dumont (1970) translates Talcott Parsons has relevance for what I am suggesting here: "To adopt a value is to introduce hierarchy, and a certain consensus of values, a certain hierarchy of ideas, things and people, is indispensable to social life" (20). Value, he seems to say in the first part of this sentence, entails hierarchy; something or someone is inevitably valued more or less than something or someone else. Most of the time the carriers of a certain set of values may not realize this, but at times, the ways in which some values are less important than others becomes apparent. Dumont also asserts the necessity of a degree of value consensus for social cohesion. Numbulwar, however, may not be a site best characterized in this way. From my perspective, it is a place where there are at least two, more or less shared, socially and historically patterned hierarchies of value, one for blackfellas and one for white-fellas, that in ordering what matters only sometimes overlap.

Oriented as I am by a perspective derived from schema theory, I assume that values are internalized as components of schema that, working in concert with other schema content, create our sense of not only how the world is but also how it should be (Strauss and Quinn 1997:94). Hence values, while becoming conscious only in some circumstances, are motivational in all.[25] The, at least temporary, resilience and impermeability of a value hierarchy and the potential it has for generating if not conflict then surprise or confusion in intercultural settings may be seen in the following brief account of the new shop at Numbulwar.

Thursday September 4, 2003, Numbulwar

Around 10:10 AM Went to office and shop…Ran into Lily and went with her to shop, new, on opposite side of road from old one which has been torn down except steel skeleton. (2003:I:12)

While this journal entry introduces the appearance of the new shop, it does not capture my sense of dislocation and confusion upon finding the shop located where I did on my first visit to Numbulwar's town center in 2003. In 1997, I had found it in what looked like a new building on the other side of the road. Was my memory at fault? Maybe the steel skeleton was the old Council building; maybe the shop had always been located across the road? Over time, I learned that my memory was not the problem. The relatively new shop of 1997 had subsequently been "cursed" by what was once referred to as an "old man," though more recently as a "clan" or even "tribal" "elder," a man seen to have considerable ritual power. This man refused to remove the curse, and since no one senior in the ritual hierarchy was willing to make the shop a safe place again, a new shop was built across the road, while the old one was dismantled and carted off to the rubbish tip. Until the new shop's construction was complete, people were able to do their shopping in the recreation hall.

Ever since I have been visiting Numbulwar, people have been cursing other people or places or things. An expression of displeasure and anger that generally has the effect of intimidating others, cursing was usually, but not exclusively, performed by men. When something was cursed, it was "put"—a simple verbal act—to a ceremony, sacred place, or dead person. This need not be done by a person who was present, and drinkers from as far away as Borroloola or Nhulunbuy have been known to send a telegram or ring up to tell someone that somebody or something at Numbulwar has been cursed. When the sacred or the dead is put to something, rules applying to the sacred and the dead also apply, that is, the person, place, or object became sacred, dangerous, and to be avoided until the curse is removed (Burbank 1994:35–6, 168–70; see also O'Donnell 2007:68:ff42,28:ff28). In the case of the shop, the sacred clearly trumped a substantial building in a value hierarchy. I leave it to readers to think of cases where the sacred so trumps the material in Western experience.

My task here is to render this act at least somewhat intelligible for anyone who may marvel at a decision to discard material worth thousands of dollars in a community always strapped for resources, "simply," from a whitefella perspective, because it had been cursed. While I agree with others (e.g., Shore 1996) that cultural accounts alone are insufficient to explain human action (288), we move toward understanding with a discussion of the relative value, in a blackfella hierarchy, of material goods on the one hand, and relationships, at least those that both whitefellas and blackfellas would call particularly "close" ones, on the other.

> [A man] bought some batteries for that new tape recorder. And he was fixing it and [his three-year old grandson] was there and [the man] told him, "Don't push all the buttons." And his grandson just dropped the tape recorder [from about 2 feet off the ground] and went away. So [the man] picked up the tape and went to the toilet and you know that round bowl, he just smashed the tape against it and smashed it again and again. And his son came but he was too late, the tape recorder was finished. And [his grandson] didn't stay with [his grandmother and grandfather] that night. (Aboriginal speaker in Burbank 1994:153–4)

Over the years that I have been visiting Numbulwar, incidents such as this one have come to my attention on many occasions. The items destroyed have varied; instead of a tape recorder they might be an electric kettle, the windshield of a vehicle, or the outdoor lights surrounding the basketball court. So too have the relationships of the protagonists varied; they might, for example, be several brothers, or sisters, a pair of lovers, a mother and her adult children, or, rarely, an Aboriginal person and a whitefella superordinate. Sometimes the destruction of an item accompanies an act of physical aggression directed at another person such as striking out with a fighting stick or a broom. Yet, even when direct interpersonal physical aggression was not part of the action, people often used words such as "fight" and its Wubuy translation *wungarri* in their telling of such events.

The destruction of property as a means of resolving tensions between kin has been duly noted in the ethnography of Aboriginal Australia. As an example almost as dramatic as the dismantled shop, Sutton (2009) remarks on a case where a house was burned down (81); Myers (1988) mentions that more than one Pintupi vehicle has been set alight to this end (61). In past analyses of indirect physical aggression (Burbank 1985; 1994:151–5), I have suggested that attacks on objects may be understood as displacement behaviors (Freud 1989; Dollard et al. 1969). Rather than "kill," that is, strike, a person, people at Numbulwar kill objects. It seems clear that it is the value of specific relationships that redirects people's violence toward less valued targets, often material things. Though cast in the language of a "structural interpretation," W. Lloyd Warner (1937) came to a similar conclusion about aggressive acts associated with *mirriri*, the masculine response to a breach of the etiquette required by the adult brother/sister relationship.[26] In Yolngu speaking parts of Arnhem Land, as at Numbulwar, this consisted of throwing spears at any sister present:

> The interpretation is simple. Her patrilineal and family bond are very strong; everyone knows that in a final test a brother would fight his own dué [brother-in-law] if he went too far when mistreating her. Given the fact that a man cannot hear his sister sworn at, he must choose either to defend his sister and fight her husband, or do nothing. If he chose the first, it would immediately endanger and possibly destroy for the time the whole lateral structure of his clan's kinship with the rest of the tribe...Doing nothing is conceivable, but extremely difficult if the emotions are highly aroused by the mirriri. It is out of keeping with general Murngin behaviour not to express an emotion socially. Therefore an entirely different possibility has been seized upon and socialized. The sister is treated as though she were her husband, and spears are thrown at her as though she and not he were the culprit. This saves any trouble between the clans. (Warner 1937:100–101)

Given Warner's supposition (or perhaps it was an observation) that a sister would not be seriously injured by such an act, we can imagine her occupying a place similar to that of an object, at least in a "brother's" mind. In these acts, angry people are able to give expression to their feelings in an expected manner without harming others, at least physically, and endangering valued relationships, at least not to the extent they might should they directly attack a person (Burbank 1994). It is not, perhaps, so much the monetary cost of items damaged and destroyed in these affairs, as the desires people display to own or use them, and the difficulties they may have in obtaining them, that underline the greater value placed upon specific relationships. These are usually those of family.

Family

Divergent understanding in intercultural circumstances does not simply arise from different language competencies. Talking with people in this community means being with people, though what can only be described as an explosion of mobile phone use during the study period might presage more disembodied forms of interaction. For the most part, non-Indigenous residents spent their time with spouses, colleagues, clients, and friends; Aboriginal people spent their time with kin, particularly "family," a word used by Aboriginal people at Numbulwar to talk about what anthropologists call a kindred, that is, "an egocentrically defined field of close kin" (Shapiro 1981:41), or a segment of the kindred, such as a woman's children. Individuals within the kindred might also be referred to as family, as in, "He is my family" or "those two boys are my families."

Sometimes a person would be described as "close family." It would appear that, like whitefellas, blackfellas employ spatial metaphors to distinguish between kin; here "close" indicates not only the perception of a more direct genealogical connection[27] between people but also the possibility that the relationship is one of greater intimacy. Consonant with this conceptualization of relationship was the effort I saw family make to maintain psychological if not actual physical proximity to each other.[28] For example, mobile phones were programed almost exclusively with other family members' numbers and used predominantly to phone them; current and planned whereabouts were often the topics of conversation.

The degree to which family may be close at Numbulwar, however, likely surpasses much in the experience of "closeness" for many whitefellas. Family are not simply close but, in some cases or in some ways, interchangeable.

•

V: What kind of punishment did they have for young men who did not follow the rules?

AM: What usually happened, they either get speared in the traditional way, if they don't watch what they do, even if they do small things, pinch something, they get speared. Everybody, the whole clan's gotta fight this bloke and makem realize what he did. After he will be told, because he has broken the Law told to him in the ceremony place, that's gonna cost him and his family their lives. That's how strict it is. He has to think of a way to save himself and his family. Make a payment in public with all the Law people, pay for his family's life. All the family come together. If he don't do that, slowly the family will be disintegrated. Until they leave the last person of that family. (Senior male speaker in Burbank 2006:10)

This man is, of course, referring to what must be understood as a largely imagined past. As will be seen in later chapters, however, the near identity of family members that the speaker portrays, and hence must be regarded as an aspect of his subjectivity, was also quite apparent in talk about sorcery, thought to be a widespread activity during the years of the study.

Sharing and not sharing, as will be seen in chapter four, are highly relevant concerns when it comes to family:

> Family, we family, we give each other everything. If my family have no anything, I give them flour, sugar, baking powder, smoke [cigarettes] or sometime I go to my sister's place; they give me dugong when my sister's husband go hunting or they cooking turtle. We share everything to our kids, show them how to share. And the other family, we look after each other like [clan name] mob, [clan name] mob. I look after a lot of people. I give a lot to people. They ask me for money, I don't say no. I don't say, "Go away from my house." I invite people to come in. We sit and tell each other story like Dreamtime story. Or you go to other people's house, sit down, have a yarn, that's a family. (Emma 2005)

Children do indeed seem to be prepared for a life of sharing as many recorders of Aboriginal life have noted. Sitting one day with a family group outside the church for a funeral held in 2005, I watched a girl, about ten years of age, take a peanut she had already placed in her mouth, the last one in the packet, and give it to a toddler who, watching her eat, had said, "peanut." Following the toddler's experience of being given a peanut when he asked for, or simply noticed it, he in turn was asked by one of his adult female kin for some of his soft drink, "Give me some uncle." His mother said, "Give your *marig* [kin reciprocal of uncle] some," and he offered the bottle to her, an example of the kind of socialization practice and child response I have seen repeatedly over the years.

When I invited Kay, a woman I have known since her adolescence, to come stay with me in Perth, I mentioned she would have to share a bathroom. "That's alright," she joked, "I am blackfella, we share everything." For Aboriginal people across Australia, sharing "emerges repeatedly in the ways Aboriginal people define themselves" (Peterson and Taylor 2003:107–108). In the earlier quote, Emma defined family as people who "give each other everything," people who "share everything." During the years of the study, Emma attended a course in Indigenous studies in which she might have heard versions of the statement that "caring and sharing [are] the first two rules of Aboriginality" (Gilbert 1978:304–305 in ibid., 108), a further, though only imagined, example of intercultural possibilities. Whether or not this is so, her emphasis on "sharing" in response to a question about family suggests an important connection between ideas and feelings about family and about being an Aboriginal person. Most pertinent here, sharing everything might be seen as a practice that differentiates whitefellas from blackfellas.

The role that sharing plays in whitefella/blackfella differentiation as a patterned component of Aboriginal identity and hence of Aboriginal culture was also noted by at least one of the whitefellas that I interviewed: "I'll give food or something to someone and others say 'friend,' 'cus' [Kriol kin term]. It means they want some. Sharing is very strong. They don't think we share, we're very selfish people. And we are, except that we have a mortgage" (ITU 2004). In my experience, it is only by being "adopted" into an Aboriginal family that social intercourse between blackfellas and whitefellas becomes truly possible. Here a schoolteacher speaks about this process as she experienced it shortly after her arrival at Numbulwar:

> We're adopted at school, from [a woman]. From [the Aboriginal School Principal]. When she was here and we were starting a meeting, she said to everyone, "I'd like you all to go into your family groups." And there we were standing alone, [another new teacher] and me and [the Principal] said, "How do these people feel, no family?" (ITU 2005)

While it probably is a comfort to the new whitefella to receive a kin status, as appears to have been the Nunggubuyu School principal's intention, we might consider that the comfort is felt on both sides. It is not merely a question of facilitating social etiquette. Sustained and meaningful interaction needs to take place with kin. One whitefella present at Numbulwar during this study did not wish to be categorized as anyone's kinsperson, feeling that such a label would interfere with her ability to do her job, a preference she, no doubt, made known. Gradually, however, people began to call her by a variety of kin terms. As best I can tell, these were consonant with the identity of a single focal ego, though an Aboriginal person as a fictive kinsperson was never named, and perhaps did not exist. It is worth mentioning here that one of my granddaughters used the word "find," as in "How did [my fictive sister] find you?" when asking me how I became her grandmother. Find is a word used to signify parenthood, usually to speak of a man fathering a child. Its use here, I believe, calls attention to my adoption both as an achievement and a reality, a position that might be contrasted to the anthropological use of "fictive." What may be the considerable emotional importance of these relationships was first underlined years ago when a school teacher told me that she had changed her clan and thus kin relationship with the woman who had originally volunteered (or had been chosen to volunteer) to be her sister. She needed, as a part of her job, to interact with a man who was, according to her original kin status, her son-in-law and thus to be avoided, as the etiquette of this relationship would dictate. However reasonable whitefellas might find her justification for making this change, the now ex-sister refused to speak to her.

Even without having one's relationship rejected, it is likely that, from an Aboriginal perspective, whitefellas make "strange kin," to slightly reword a phrase from Redmond (2005). Numerous observers of Aboriginal Australia have found that blackfellas make use of whitefellas to deflect demands or escape from obligations in a manner reminiscent of what Myers (1986) has described as the use of the Dreaming in Pintupi social life. There, tensions between the priority of family relatedness and a disinclination to either limit one's own or another's autonomy were once, and perhaps continue to be, surmounted by deference to the sacred, an authority located outside the immediacy of kin. More recently, Pintupi found that authority vested in a "white boss" provided a similar solution (Myers 1986). Redmond (2005) tells of a pastoralist with a history of intercultural interaction that implicated him in the moral economy of local Ngarinyin people; his marriage to a "Euro-Australian wife" "came to act as a partial foil against demand sharing" (240). Peterson and Taylor (2003) likewise see non-Indigenous partners in marriages with Indigenous people, usually women, providing the "acceptable grounds for deflecting demands." Brady (1995, in Peterson and Taylor 2003:114) tells of Aboriginal people using the authority of whitefella doctors to justify their disinclination to join groups of drinkers. I have long been asked by my family to store precious items such as tape recorders and tobacco, and instructed to refuse should I be asked for them by others.

When my family cast me in such a role, however, what are they saying about me? It might be that, to use Redmond's (2005:239) alternatives, they simply perceived me to be a more distant kind of kin and thus more able to refuse the demands they anticipate from others. It could be, however, that I am seen to have a "hard chest," or to use the language of a Numbulwar perhaps somewhat past, a "strong *binji*" [guts/abdomen]. It strikes me as highly plausible that whitefellas like me provide important information to Aboriginal people about the whitefella world, including how to be in the whitefella world of things. One piece of information may be that whitefellas are better able than blackfellas to acquire and keep things; in particular, we are better able to resist sharing with our family (cf. Austin-Broos 2009:130).

Value Conflict

NUD: Turnover is very high. The average stay [of whitefellas] would be about one year, probably less than that.

VKB: What do you think are the reasons for the high turnover?

NUD: Remoteness, frustration with trying to get a job done and always being thwarted.

VKB: What thwarts people?

NUD: Cultural difference. Aboriginal people don't turn up to work and when they do they don't take responsibility for what they do. That really gets to some people. A whitefella is usually a manager, and is asked by the granting body that funds the work, to work to a certain standard which is not realistic given the circumstances here. There is a conflict between outside expectations and what the person can do, given available resources and human resources. I would say frustration like this is number one reason for leaving. (NUD 2003)

In chapter six, I will suggest that Numbulwar's Aboriginal people don't "turn up" because they give priority to family matters that may compete or conflict with whitefella activities and arrangement. In chapter four, I delineate what I see as the emotional source of this priority, a highly responsive form of early childrearing. "Cultural difference," the divergence of blackfella and whitefella experiences, particularly of whitefella practices and institutions, appears to rest on the priority that family relationships are given in a blackfella hierarchy of value (see also Austin-Broos 2009; Myers 1986; 1988).

To speak, however, of just one hierarchy of value for whitefellas and one for blackfellas is likely a distortion (see also Robbins 2007; Shore 1996:284–302). If we understand "value" and value hierarchy to be premised on mental schema, we can understand the potential that values, and the ways in which they are ordered, have to change, not simply in a person's lifetime, but in a given set of circumstances in that lifetime. The extent to which whitefellas and blackfellas have learned values from each other must remain an open question here but clearly individuals learn from their cross-cultural encounters. I imagine, for example, that prior to her experience at Numbulwar,

the whitefella schoolteacher speaking earlier would not have so readily described herself as "selfish" in the way she does in that quote. It
is also clear that Aboriginal people have learned to value many items
and arrangements from the West. The question then becomes not one
of shared values, but of shared priorities. Both whitefellas and blackfellas may care about relationships and material resources, but the
different places these values appear to occupy in their respective value
hierarchies undoubtedly underlie the observable patterns of difference
in decisions made and actions taken. If we accept that values are associated with a way of life, that is, a way of staying alive if not flourishing (Vogt and Albert 1966a), it is not surprising that whitefella and
blackfella priorities diverge. Whitefellas, after all, do have to pay a
mortgage, and blackfellas have little to rely on beside their family.

Some whitefellas, however, have paid off their mortgage, or never
had one, and some blackfellas don't have much of a family on which
to rely. I have long noted that some Aboriginal people "turn up" at
school and work much more regularly than others. Some of these
are people whose family circumstances might be described as less
than ideal, for example, people who have experienced a mother's
death or a father's desertion in their childhood. Myers (1986) has
observed that Pintupi orphans and children who have lost a parent
are most likely to become petrol sniffers. In contrast, I find his conclusion that "their...attitude attempts to build a self-reliance in the
face of devastating loss" (178) consonant with my observation that
it is sometimes just such people who come to value extra-familial
Western institutions over family, the impersonal over the familial,
and act in terms of this ordering.

It is not simply socially disadvantaged blackfellas who may
have been coming to value the material over the personal, however. I have long observed fights and arguments over material items
(e.g., Burbank 1994); similar events took place between 2003 and
2005, some of which will be presented in later chapters. Nor should
the importance of family be interpreted to mean that Numbulwar is
one big happy family.

> VKB: Who wanted you to send [a man, , who had been walking
> around the community armed with spears, proclaiming his sor-
> row, anger and suspicions of foul play, following the death of a
> kinsman] away?
> TOT: [Several senior Aboriginal people] and all the *balanda*
> [whitefella].[29] There was a lot of pressure on me. This is common
> when anyone is causing trouble. People come to me and ask, "Can

you send him away?" "No!" I answer. It was a constant comment, a general comment whenever [the man] was yelling up at the shop. "Oh we're sick of this. It will be your fault if he kills someone." [A senior Aboriginal man] was most vocal. I said, "I can't send him away, ring the police." Finally I said, "Unless you are willing to come with me to the police, I can't do anything." That stopped them because nobody was willing to call the police. (TOT 2004)

In chapters four and five, experiences that represent less a clear hierarchy of value than what may be a conflict of values are presented in discussions of stress, "black magic" (i.e., sorcery), and identity. In the next chapter, I continue this introduction to Numbulwar and its people though an interpretation of a more distant past via a fetal origins of health and disease model.

Chapter 3

Life History and Real Life: Fetal Origins of Disease, Ethnography, and History

Models

The relentless procession of illness, disability, death, and grief manifest at Numbulwar in recent years has compelled me to ask how this has happened to people whom I once saw as so vital. When and where did this plague of ill health begin? In a study where health and departures from health are major themes, it seems particularly important, but also difficult, to identify relevant but not obvious factors (Farmer 2004). Ethnographers primarily concerned with the here and now of participant observation nevertheless find it necessary to include less visible, less immediate information in their portrayals of the human condition; they routinely incorporate historical material in their accounts. In the field of Indigenous Australia, the injustices of colonization have been highlighted by anthropologists and others addressing issues of health inequality (e.g., Carson et al. 2007; Reid and Lupton 1991:xii; Saggers and Grey 1991). History, though, is just as multifaceted as ethnography. On what basis can we identify components of the past that are most germane for a current portrayal? And how are we to understand the extra-personal processes and structures that interpenetrate people's real life experience, in this case experiences of ill health and death? Just how does the destruction of a way of life create a legacy of premature morbidity and mortality? This is where models come in. In this chapter, as is also customary in much of anthropology, I move across disciplines for these, in line with the general orientation of this work, to the biological and medical sciences.

It has been suggested that our view of "health as a single, attainable, and sustainable state may be a heuristic, but ultimately unrealistic, concept" (Ellison 2005:118). In place of the dichotomous health/disease framework this view implies, we might alternatively understand health as a series of ongoing tradeoffs required of organisms by their circumstances. This perspective enables a view of Indigenous health where pathology is ascribed not so much to physiology as to environment. In taking this position I am guided by recent conceptual reworkings of what is known variously as the "Barker hypothesis," "the fetal origins of disease" model and "the developmental origins of health and disease" model. This reconceptualization places it within a life history framework, and invites us to consider the mechanisms of our species' life history strategies (Ellison 2005; Worthman and Kuzara 2005).

This formulation of the fetal origins of disease hypothesis allows me to circumvent a nature/nurture form of dichotomization found sometimes in the social determinants of health arena. For example, Gray et al. (2004) present the Barker hypothesis as an alternative to "the social exclusion" hypothesis (Executive Summary:1). In contrast, the perspective I present grounds this discussion of Numbulwar's history both in the social and the physiological. It becomes possible for us to see "social exclusion," for example, as a possible precursor of maternal constraint, a physiological factor (discussed in the following pages) that may contribute to later experiences of socially generated stress. This approach focuses our attention on aspects of the environment that stress mothers and, later, their offspring, whether such aspects be physical or social. It also allows us to consider the manner in which environmental stressors may have intergenerational consequence for health.

Fetal Origins

Human life history, that is, our species-specific pattern of birth, development, reproduction, and death, may be characterized as prolonged and plastic (e.g., Bateson and Martin 2000; Worthman 1999). An example of our plasticity may be seen in the fetal capacity to adapt to the uterine environment by modifying its rate and type of growth. Evidence suggests that when a fetus is undernourished, the placental blood supply is directed away from some developing organs to others. Thus, depending on gestational period, blood might be directed away from the developing kidneys to the brain, that supremely vital human structure. This individual's kidneys are likely to have fewer cells than those of a fetus better nourished during development; and kidneys with fewer cells are more likely to fail if stressed later on (Barker 1994:123).

As this example foreshadows, plasticity has its costs. It necessarily leads to what have been thought to be permanent changes in individual physiology, though recently this view has been challenged (e.g., Gunnar and Quevedo 2007:163; Wyrwoll et al. 2006). These changes may contribute to a greater disease burden in later life. Low birth weight (i.e., a less than expected newborn weight) has become the index of this future cost. Forms of adult ill health associated with low birth weight include coronary heart disease, stroke, hypertension, type 2 diabetes (and obesity in association with this condition), depressive disorders, and schizophrenia (Barker 2004; Ericksson et al. 2003; Thompson et al. 2001; Wahlbeck et al. 2001). All these conditions are found at Numbulwar.

Low birth weight, characteristic of a number of children (Burbank and Chisholm 1989), is seen in the model I draw upon as a consequence of uterine environments where resources are restricted or unpredictable. These kinds of uterine environment are seen, in turn, as the consequence of "poor or uncertain maternal nutrition, poor maternal health, and/or high allostatic load" (Worthman and Kuzara 2005:98). Allostatic load is what we call "stress," the cumulative biological cost of maintaining stability vis-à-vis changes in internal and external environments (McEwen and Wingfield 2003). While nutrients in the placental blood supply may be what the fetal-placental unit responds to, more than maternal nutritional status may be responsible for this state (Gluckman et al. 2007:8–10). The experience of social stress, such as inequality and injustice, may, in and of itself, diminish a woman's capacity to nourish her fetus in spite of an adequate diet.

In this model the neuroendocrine architecture, particularly that of the hypothalamic-pituitary-adrenal (HPA) axis, is cast as the mechanism for implementing a human life history strategy via resource allocation. Worthman and Kuzara (2005) review an extensive literature on birth weight, stress, and health outcomes. Given the pervasive role of the neuroendocrine architecture in body composition and function, they are not surprised to find associations between a birth weight continuum and variation in organ composition and function, body composition, metabolic regulation, and functioning of components of the endocrine system. There is a greater likelihood that as low birth weight individuals develop, their bodies will contain, for example, more fat, less muscle, and fewer kidney cells than higher birth weight individuals. They are also likely to have greater resistance to insulin (105, 106). This model suggests that a consideration of the physical, social, and cultural environments in which mothers may be well or ill nourished, in good or poor health, relatively secure and happy or anxious and depressed is essential background for analyses of the current health environment. Thus, the incorporation of relevant history into this account would seem to be worthwhile.

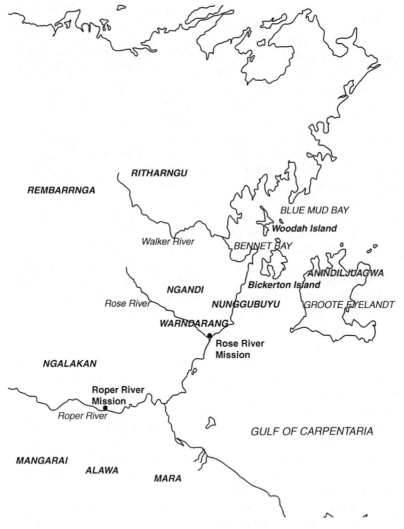

Map 3.1   Based on Heath 1978:13; Hughes 1971:i–iii.

History

Given the widespread characterization of Indigenous health as poor, however, is there a point in looking for community-specific underlying factors? The history of Indigenous Australians from 1788 onward makes it clear that regardless of the precise time of contact and nature of change, every Indigenous community in Australia has faced the potential extinction of its way of life or its people (e.g., McGrath 1995). It seems reasonable to assume a shared state of disruption leading to widespread mental and physical ill health of Indigenous people across the continent. Yet as Sutton (2009) says with reference to "Indigenous community dysfunction," "there are many regional differences within Indigenous Australia, making continent-wide generalisations difficult" (81, 82). It is in an examination of the differences, the specific perturbations encountered by different individuals in different communities, where I believe ethnography has so much to offer, enabling us to move from the level of theory to that of experience.

I begin my search with Numbulwar's past, though scant materials make this history more conjectural than I would like.[1]

Initially, the immediate ancestors of Numbulwar's contemporary population seem to have been relatively well nourished, healthy, and unstressed. For people occupying the more northern parts of Nunggubuyu lands, the pre-mission environment appears bountiful and peaceful, at least in this vignette:

> There was a big camp of the Nungubuyu Tribe on this eastern shore of Bennet Bay at this season [June, 1935], numbering approximately 100 natives—men, women and children. They had concentrated in this sheltered bay following the stormy weather that had prevailed for some time past, and were reengaged in dugong and turtle hunting...[T]he natives were very friendly, most of them had already made some contact with white men either in the camp at the mouth of the Roper River, or on visits to the missions at Groote or Roper River. Dugong and turtle fishing was carried on very industriously, and soon after sunrise each morning a fleet of five or six canoes would set out for the fishing grounds, from half a mile to a mile offshore. Other game, especially fish was very plentiful, and all the natives were well fed, and in good condition. Children were numerous in this camp. (Thomson 1936:8–9)

However, an earlier account of the Reverend Mr. H. E. Warren's visit in 1916 portrays a somewhat different state of affairs for

Nunggubuyu living to the south at the mouth of the Rose River:

> The blacks have a large camp here. At 4.30 Mr. Dyer and self each
> had a service with pictures. Umbereare and Rupert helped him, and
> Daniel and Alec assisted me. He had 34 men and I had 37 women and
> children; but we could not persuade all the natives to come and lis-
> ten. After service I dressed some half-dozen wounds—one man's leg
> dreadfully eaten away; one boy seriously ill; but I could do nothing
> for him, as he was only a few weeks old. (Cole 1982:21)

The Nunggubuyu also seem to have been spared the harsher aspects
of colonization. As far as I can tell, pre-mission contact was largely
restricted to visits from Macassan trepangers (Thomson 1983:22).
These visits may well have been stimulating and enriching encounters, if their traces in dance, loan words, and artifacts are any indication.[2] To the west, south, and north of Nunggubuyu countries,
however, Aboriginal people appear not to have been so fortunate
(Bauer 1964; Cole 1979; Merlan 1978; Morphy and Morphy 1984;
Reid 1990; Thomson 1983). It seems likely that word of social and
ecological disruption brought with the pastoral expansion in the
late 1800s might have reached as far as Nunggubuyu country. On
the other hand, the more northern Wubuy speakers may have been
buffered, at least for a while, from the fearsome sort of news others
might hear. Thomson (1983) remarked of the Nunggubuyu people
at Bennet Bay mentioned earlier that:

> The people in the camp at Bennet Bay knew nothing about the Blue
> Mud Bay people or their movements, although they lived within sight
> of Woodah Island and must frequently have seen their canoes. But the
> anomaly is explained by the fact that a distinct cultural break occurs
> just here and the Nunggubuyu cannot understand the language of
> their northern neighbours of Woodah Island and the hinterland of
> Blue Mud Bay, so that there is a minimum of contact between the two
> peoples...All the southerners [Nunggubuyu] regarded the peoples of
> the northern end of Blue Mud Bay as enemies, and were very unwill-
> ing to venture into their territory. (42)

At the time Thomson refers to, the Woodah Islanders were infa-
mous for the murders of several Japanese pearlers and Europeans.
This group of Nunggubuyu probably did learn about the Woodah
Island murders and the imprisonment of the perpetrators, if not
from Thomson then from Joshua, his guide, a Wandarang man
from Roper River Mission. It is also possible that they had heard of

this before Thomson's trip, as three CMS missionaries had under-taken what church historian Keith Cole (1982) described as "the world renowned Peace Expedition" (22–3). This trio traveled to Caledon Bay, just to the north of Woodah Island and "persuaded the Aboriginal killers of five Japanese fishermen, two white beach-combers and Constable A. S. McColl to give themselves up and go to Darwin for trial" (23).

Language barriers did not prevent the Nunggubuyu from at least second hand, if not first hand, experiences of white violence in the Rose River area and to the south. Cole (1985), for example, writing about the 1908 founding of Roper River Mission, remarked:

> The tribes in the Roper River area had been decimated by the depredations of the pastoralists, and their tribal organisation had been smashed. The main tribes in the area, and those now severely depleted, were the Mara, Alawa, Wandarang, Ngandi, Ngalakan, the southernmost members of the Rembarrnga and Nunggubuyu tribes, and some of the Mangarayi tribe. (57)

Residents at Numbulwar identify not only with Nunggubuyu but also with several other of these language groups, each with a differ-ent history of interaction with the colonial environmental. Just as their language group identities vary, so we might imagine that their stress lineages vary in their potential for intergenerational harm (see also Gunnar and Quevedo 2007:163).[3]

In August of 1952, seventeen years after Thomson's trip to Bennet Bay, the Anglican Church Missionary Society (CMS) established the Rose River Mission on what may be regarded as Nunggubuyu land, though it is said to be the country of a clan that originally spoke Wandarang (Heath 1978:13, 16). Within a week of their arrival, the Aboriginal population had increased to over one hundred men, women, and children, growing in that short time from the original sixty-five Aboriginal people who had accompanied the missionaries up the coast from Roper River Mission (Cole 1982: 2830–31).

Rose River Mission was not the first settlement experience for Nunggubuyu people. Mission histories indicate that they had a pres-ence at Roper River Mission, certainly from the 1940s onward, and as the quote presented earlier suggests, perhaps from the beginning of the Roper Mission. Similarly, Numbulwar's Anindiljuagwa speak-ers from families on Bickerton Island and Groote Eylandt may well have ancestors with a history of extended mission contact beginning in 1921, when the first CMS mission was established on the larger of the two islands (Cole 1985). Mainland people, too, may have older relatives with long experience of the Groote Island missions (e.g., Heath 1978:16; 1980:499). What factors in these new circumstances may be associated with poor nutrition, poor health, anxiety, and unhappiness?

John Mercer (1978) is identified as the missionary in charge of the first boat loads of Nunggubuyu people to be transferred from Roper River Mission to the planned site of the Rose River Mission (Cole 1981:28). In his account, this new Church Missionary Society settlement, though long a possibility, was realized because of a drought:

> In the providence of God the summer of 1951–52 in Eastern Arnhem Land turned into a severe drought. Portable water along the Roper River dried up and dysentery became rife among the various tribal groups congregated at the Roper River Mission...
>
> The Nunggubuyu people from Rose River were represented at the Roper Mission, and after a visit to the area in Mid 1952 it was recommended the section of the Nunggubuyu people camping at the mission be transferred to their own tribal lands. (Mercer 1978: Introduction)

Neither Aboriginal people nor missionaries telling me the story of Rose River Mission's establishment mentioned a drought. They emphasized the initiative of Wubuy-speaking people who desired a mission. These accounts begin with the "Mid 1952" trip to "their own tribal lands." A version of this account is included in an "anonymous history" of Numbulwar's first ten years unearthed by Cole (1982):

> After doing the survey along the Rose River and scouting inland in search of cypress pine, they spent a few days at the mouth of the river sheltering from the strong south-easterly winds which had arisen. While there Madi took Mr. Mercer to see his country and showed him the large corroboree grounds with the sacred poles and the various places where people had camped when they had gathered there for high ceremonies. While they stood there talking, he asked when the CMS was going to commence a mission at Rose River and he went on to say that the people would like it right where the sacred place was situated. (27–8)[4]

Madi, a man who had died shortly before my first visit to Numbulwar in 1977, gives his version of this account in the following segments extracted from Heath's (1980) translation[5]:

> Long ago, back in those days (when we were) in the bush. My people, we who stayed (there), I was in charge of them. We went along, I got them up and made them go (from Nunggubuyu country). We stayed (for a while) at Groote Eylandt. Things were all right, we were working (at the mission at Angurugu).
>
> Then there was a fight (between us Nunggubuyu and the Anindhilyagwa-speaking natives of Groote). We had a dispute, then they (all of us) threw spears, there was a spear fight. "How about it?" (I said to the other Nunggubuyu). I took them back (to the mainland) and we stayed in the bush.
>
> We went (for tobacco) to Roper River Mission (now Ngukurr settlement). Again we worked there, but again after a while we got into a fight. They had a spearfight, we had a spearfight. Again we came back (to our country). Along here (around Numbulwar mission) we ate dugong and sea turtles. After that, over there at the place Wurindi, we ate terrestrial game animals (birds, kangaroos and wallabies, etc.) . . .
>
> We went along, then (we stayed at) Groote Eylandt (again). Then there was a real fight, we had a (big) fight, spearing each other. One group threw spears from one side, and they (other group) were on this side. (I.e. the two opposing parties lined up opposite on another and threw spears). (499–500)

Both Aboriginal people and missionaries telling me about Numbulwar's origins mentioned the fighting that had taken place between the Nunggubuyu and others at the settlements on Groote Eylandt and at Roper River; both groups of speakers presenting it as a motive for establishing the Rose River Mission. Madi, too, appears to have seen this friction with other groups as the precipitating cause of the Nunggubuyu exodus and the founding of a settlement of their own:

> (I said) "I am going to take them (my people) away today." And I took them away (from Groote) that same day. We stayed on the beach (on the mainland). That was finished, we came from there (from Groote).
>
> When I went back there (briefly, to Groote, I spoke (about setting up a distinct mission for the Nunggubuyu).
>
> I spoke then about the (future) mission. This mission standing here at Numbulwar. I spoke about it (i.e. pleaded to have it built). The bishop arrived and I grabbed him (and pleaded with him). I kept talking about it. Mr. Montgomery arrived.

I kept speaking (pleading). (He said to me,) "How about Bickerton (Island)?" (I said,) "No! It's too small." I kept speaking. (He suggested my country (i.e. Murungun clan territory around Cape Barrow). (I said,) "No! The water supply is bad (just a lot of) muddy water." I kept speaking. (He said,) "(How about) the place Dharari." "All right, Dharari."

This mission here (at Numbulwar), this one here, was going to be at that place Dharari. (However,) after that we came (i.e. we just kept going) down around here. The words (a message) were waiting for me.

...

"Your mission (i.e. building material for mission, etc.) is ready. Take it!" All of these things I took... "Your mission is ready, here is your shed and your kitchen." (502–504)

The Aboriginal agency apparent in these accounts is belied, however, by much of what appears to have taken place during the mission years. Then, in accordance with the Commonwealth's Assimilation Policy, missionaries or other Westerners were in charge of the store, school, health clinic, church, and the basic governance of Rose River Mission (Cole 1982; Young 1981). That the Mission was run in an authoritarian fashion is implied by Cole (1982) when he describes "mission discipline" as "strict," providing the following example from the journal of John Mercer: "Sunday 31.8.52...During the afternoon I had to request that a corroboree be discontinued. This will prove a helpful illustration to tomorrow's address on the fourth commandment" (30). The extent of mission control in the early decades of Rose River Mission is suggested in the following:

From June 1967 the catering for children was gradually phased out. Up till that time the children had been fed and given school clothes. The teacher at school had supervised showers, teeth cleaning, clothes changes and meals. The clothes had been washed by school laundresses and the older children had helped with serving and washing-up at meal times. As has been mentioned the system came under increased scrutiny by the missionaries. *They now decided that the parents should be given the responsibility* of washing and mending school clothes, and a greater part in providing meals. (54; My emphasis)

Control was also exerted indirectly via the services provided on the mission. For example, here is an excerpt from the 1966 Annual Report: "Only wholemeal flour was used in cooking and sold in the shop. The sale of sugar, biscuits and sweets is still restricted" (in Cole 1982:53). The subordination of Aboriginal people by these forms of control was likely accompanied and exacerbated by the "Europeans'" attitudes toward Indigenous people. Cole (1979) captures something of what this might have been when he discusses the CMS missions for "half caste" children in the Northern Territory during his period:

> Changes in community attitudes to part-Aborigines has been a feature of the past seventy years. In the early days men and women of compassion cared and acted while the white community despised and governments remained indifferent. Human bodies as well as human souls mattered to them. These people of compassion did what they thought was right. They took them away from meddling whites and unwholesome blacks, and taught them the "better" way of the white man. (132)

It was also control not welcome by at least some if not all Aboriginal people:

> A little later I looked out from my window down toward the garden and there was this amazing sight again of the two feet growing out of the base of the paper-bark tree. I said to myself : "I must go down again; perhaps I can see this wonderful thing close up." This time the aboriginal men did not warn the lazy one that I was coming. They had done that before! But now they left [the nickname of an Aboriginal man] sound asleep at the base of the paper-bark tree. So when I came down, there was [the man], fast asleep. I touched his shoulder. He woke immediately and jumped up! He had been caught out!
>
> I said, "What's the matter [nickname]? Are you tired?"
>
> He replied: "What's the matter you? You think I motor truck? All the time work, work, work, work, work!" (Mercer 1978:5)

Along with control by dominant others, the initial Aboriginal inhabitants of Rose River Mission, not to mention their descendents, were likely to have been controlled by their new physical surroundings, particularly by their houses and their spatial arrangement (Reser 1979; Sutton 2009). Reser (1979) conducted a fifteen-month field study of a remote Arnhem Land community and its outstations. Focusing on environmental control, which he links to stress, he suggests that "felt" "loss of control" and "learned helplessness" may accompany the shift from living in hunter-gather styled camps to living in Western styled houses. A house presents its inhabitants with material constraints that may or may not reflect and support valued

social arrangements. These new structures may interfere with privacy
and with etiquette (such as the *mirriri* or mother-in-law/son-in-law
avoidance). They may prevent the inclusion of those who might be
welcome intimates, and enable others less welcome to nevertheless
intrude. This latter circumstance was exacerbated at Numbulwar,
as well as on other mission and government settlements, by routine
house inspections. One mission woman, whose job it was to con-
duct them, told me of her relief when the mission abandoned this
practice.

The houses of Numbulwar past, and, perhaps, present may be
described as structures ill suited to the needs of their users. Houses
and their furnishings deteriorated rapidly because social expectations about co-residence were not matched by their design, the materials from which they were constructed did not hold up well in the
tropical costal climate, and tradespeople were too few to meet the
demand for their services. In conditions such as these, says Reser
(1979), people are repeatedly confronted by situations that require
a response beyond their capabilities (69). People forced to live in the
shabby, unsanitary, and sometimes dangerous conditions that are
generated by broken windows, exposed electrical wires, and blocked
toilets may also be living with daily reminders of their own inad-
equacy. Yet how many of us know how to replace a window, rewire
an electrical appliance, or unplug a toilet?

There are, however, indications that at Numbulwar Aboriginal
people managed to wrest back some control of their physical environment. Biernoff (1979), for example, discusses the "alien spatial
environment" of "the Village" but says:

> Despite the physical nature and constraints of Numbulwar, tra-
> ditional patterns of residence persisted. Family, lineage and clan
> areas could all be identified and patterns of social interaction related
> to them still continued...Spatially, houses were occupied in such a
> way that traditional residence patterns were paralleled remarkably
> closely, despite the fact that they were set out in rows along the two
> roads. (170)

Indeed, we may say that the original layout of Rose River Mission
reflected Aboriginal values and priorities, at least to some extent, if
it is indeed the case that Madi designed it:

> It (Cora) [a mission boat] returned. There at Wadangaja Creek we
> stayed, I stayed there.
>
> They shouted to me. I went along behind it (Cora), and there I marked

it (place). I marked out the mission area (where the missionaries lived and where the communal buildings were), and the people area (residential area for Aboriginals). I established (laid down) that. (Heath 1980:506)

With reference to this original plan, Heath remarks that "Numbulwar is still basically laid out as it was originally established in 1952" (ibid.). Biernoff (1979) notes, in addition, that people might leave their houses to camp on the beach when the weather was pleasant or when it was so hot that the ocean breeze did not cool their dwellings. I have known people to camp on the beach when the noise of amplified music has been too much for them to bear. By leaving their houses people have been able to reclaim the flexibility of the hunter-gatherer's camp, to some extent.

Relative Poverty

Another postulated source of harmful stress is relative poverty (Kawachi and Kennedy 2003; Wilkinson 1996). It is not so much "feeling poor" as "feeling poorer than others" that is implicated in ill health (Sapolsky 2004:410). It follows that the material circumstances of Aboriginal people, experienced in the context of the relative wealth of the missionaries, may have exacerbated the stressful quality of settlement life. As an example of this, we might understand that in addition to the direct effects of shoddy and inadequate shelter on physical health (Bailie 2007) and on a subjective sense of control (Reser 1979), the perception that one is not housed as well as others, may in itself be stressful.

It seems highly likely that Western styled housing and settlement layouts have had negative consequences for the social life and sense of self of Aboriginal people at Numbulwar, or at least they did so in past times (Biernoff 1979; Reser 1979). Why then, in 1977, did a woman tell me, with considerable feeling, that she wanted a "house," and why did she want a house when she was already living in one? What did she mean? The Reverend J. B. Montgomerie's 1954 annual report includes the following: "According to the Native Affairs Branch we have made much more progress at Rose River than they had anticipated...already a very good dwelling has been erected for the missionary in charge" (in Cole 1982:34). Yet houses for Aboriginal people are not mentioned until 1957: "Timber is now being cut for six native cottages. Again the native men have been taught building and carpentry, and much of the erection of the building has been done by them" (37). As Young has pointed out, the houses built for Aboriginal people compared poorly with those built for the missionaries. Writing about the housing situation in 1972, Biernoff (1979) described the "38 houses" for Aboriginal people as "inadequate by European standards" (169). Many of these were still in use during my early field trips in 1977–1978 and 1981. These small wooden structures arranged closely together in regimented rows afforded little more than shelter from rain and wind. By the time of my visits, some were wired for electricity, but none had kitchens or plumbing. In contrast, the mission houses that remained from those early years were much larger structures consisting of several rooms, including kitchens. Laundries, toilets, and showers were situated nearby.

I see this contrast in housing type as a clear example of the kind of inequality that has long been present at Numbulwar. Keeping in mind the possibility of culturally patterned variation in experience, however, I must ask if Aboriginal people at the Rose River Mission saw their housing as "inadequate" as well. More specifically, did they and if so how did they experience what I see as their relative poverty, and was this a stressful experience?[6]

By the late 1970s there is evidence of both perceptions of inequality and feelings of resentment for at least some people: "During the 1970s two blocks of conventional European style tropical houses...have been built for Aborigines. This project...was undertaken because of complaints from Aborigines that the contrast between their own living standards and those of the European residents was too great" (Young 1981:181). Musharbash (2008) has argued that houses have become a powerful metaphor of intercultural relations for the Walbiri of Yuendumu; they symbolize, simultaneously, Walbiri exclusion from the larger society and stand as a promise of future equality in that same society. Along similar lines, Gerrard (1989) has suggested that Aboriginal attempts to control the use of "European" owned or controlled vehicles in an Arnhem Land remote community reflect, at least in part, the importance of vehicles as a synecdoche of "the European collectivity, and the power that collectivity wields" (106). Myths of the "wild blackfellow," recorded by Morphy and Morphy (1984) from people in the Roper Valley, suggest that houses may be seen in a similar way by other Aboriginal groups. These stories were used by Aboriginal people who worked on the cattle stations to distinguish themselves from "wild blackfellows," Aboriginal people who were killed less than one hundred years ago in the "pacification process." In these stories, "wild blackfellows" are defined by their lack of knowledge and material wealth. Here is an excerpt from one version: "This country had loin-cloth people, or Aborigines. They had loin-cloths, nothing else, no trousers, just loin-cloths...*And they had little shelters, paperbark shelters, and they lived there, the Aborigines*" (Old Blutja in Morphy and Morphy 1984:465; My emphasis). We may at least speculate that demands for housing at Numbulwar were also demands, if not to wield the power of the missionaries, then at least to be free of its coercive force.[7]

Strong Culture, Strong Babies

Assaults on women's ability to deliver sufficient nutrients to their fetuses may have occurred in more circuitous ways as well. Many of Numbulwar's residents are the children, grandchildren, or great grandchildren of polygynists (Chisholm and Burbank 1991). From the turn of the last century, missionaries in the area opposed this marriage form—along with the premenarcheal marriage age and practice of infant betrothal associated with it—and through a concerted and sustained campaign greatly reduced its practice (Burbank 1988).

According to Cole (1977), CMS missionaries had long been concerned about the practice of polygyny, though it was not a concern they felt able to address until relatively late in mission history: "Mission pressures for (what they perceived to be) a more equitable distribution of women mainly to provide wives for unmarried men and so lessen fighting and quarrelling over women, were not felt to any great extent during the period 1908–1939" (192). While the campaign against polygyny began at the first CMS mission at Roper River, according to a missionary present in the early days of Rose River Mission, it may be that activities at the Angurugu Mission on Groote Eylandt had the most immediate effect on marriage practices at Numbulwar (Burbank 1988:62). Describing mission initiatives at Groote Eylandt, Turner (1974) says:

> In the period between 1944 and 1947...seven men belonging to Bickerton local groups who were married polygynously surrendered a total of eight wives to eight single Bickerton men. Another man gave up a wife, but after she had been married to the recipient, he reclaimed and kept her. (51)

Lily, who was a child at the time, living at Angurugu, remembers the redistribution:

> The missionary took those wives from those old men with three or four and gave them to other men. Some of the men got angry. One tried to cut him with a tommy hawk. [My mother] helped him give those women. Some stayed, some didn't. He gave [my auntie]. He gave the men tobacco, flour, tommy hawks. (Burbank 1988:62)

At Numbulwar, there was no formal redistribution of wives. However, the Aboriginal inhabitants of the mission were informed that polygyny was not consistent with a Christian way of life. And indeed, those that I have spoken with on the topic of polygyny attribute its demise to the mission, though not always to the mission's policy of "one man, one wife." One woman told me, for example, that once they were living at the mission, some women simply left their husbands. Of course, if the missionaries felt as compelled to provide "sanctuary" to such women as they were to girls under the age of sixteen who were unwilling to go to their betrothed husbands, they may well have made such acts possible (61–6).

By 2003, with only one or two exceptions, marriages were monogamous. While the preponderance of monogamy in spite of men's continuing attempts to take additional wives suggests not only women's preference for this marriage form but also their ability to maintain it in their unions, their triumph may nevertheless be another source of the ill health characteristic of contemporary times. In a monogamous marriage, one woman may have to bear the reproductive load once borne by several. For at least a time in the recent past, some women have had more children at shorter intervals than did their mothers and grandmothers.

Mercer's (1978) stories about the very early years of Rose River Mission, include mention of the expected birth spacing:

> She should not have another baby whilst she was presently nursing a child, not yet walking or able to fend for itself. So you found that aboriginal children were about three years apart in age for mothers fed their babies for two years and they reached three years before they were able to fend for themselves. (45)

Genealogies, mission and health records allowing for comparison of birth averages of 31 polygynously and 41 monogamously married women show a significantly greater number for the monogamous group, 6.05 children compared to 4.61. They also show a significant decrease, from 65.3 to 39.76 months, in the mean interbirth interval for them (Chisholm and Burbank 1991:296).[8] A significant positive correlation between birth interval and birth weight in a sample of 75 children aged zero–five years in 1988 has also been found. Children born after longer intervals tended to be heavier (Burbank and Chisholm 1989:92).

Monogamy, however, need not be associated with a greater reproductive load for individual women as Western birth rates generally demonstrate. There are other factors to be considered here. A pronatalist ideology is one that may be crucial. At least during the late 1970s, this position appeared to be characteristic of men at Numbulwar:

> Some men have a wife and for three or four years she doesn't have a child. "Oh, this girl isn't having my kids. I'll get another wife." Then he marries another girl. Might be five or six months and his second wife has a baby. She is going to have a child so she can make a race and a big family. They see when they get old, see their wife having no children. "I'll have to get another." (Aboriginal woman in Burbank 1980:104–105)

Several reasons that men might want to have children are suggested by this speaker. First among these might be the expectation that children will care for an elderly father, a reasonable expectation given the principle of reciprocity attached to parent-child relationships (Burbank 2006). I might also note the desire for a "big family" and for a "race" expressed in this text. In 1978, a woman explained to me that when Aboriginal women leave Numbulwar and marry non-Aboriginal men, people are not happy because "it makes not enough people." That is, a woman bearing children for a non-Aboriginal man is not bearing children for an Aboriginal man at Numbulwar. The possible motive of increasing the race is a poignant one, for it reminds us of the colonial violence at the margins of Nunggubuyu lands. It is also suggestive with regard to the question of the extent to which the Nunggubuyu ancestors of people at Numbulwar were aware of this violence and passed this awareness on to younger generations. Though few speak of this, at least to me, a general awareness seems likely, especially given the connections of Numbulwar's people to Ngukurr (formerly Roper Mission) (Burbank 1994:23–4). Should such violence have been interpreted along lines suggested by use of the word race and the phrase "not enough people," that is, as genocidal, the pronatalist stance of local people would not be surprising (see also Spiro 1958:100).

There are also less speculative reasons for thinking that pronatalism has been a factor, at least until recently, in determining family size. It is noteworthy that these suggest it may originate more with men than women. In an analysis of fights occurring between 1977 and 1978 precipitated by the actions of seven men attempting to obtain additional wives, I found that four of these men's wives had no children, one had only one child, and that two others were no longer fertile; in one of these cases this was due to a woman's use of contraceptives (Burbank 1994:115). This is to say that in all of these cases, infertility might have been at least a contributing factor.[9] Conversations and interviews with thirty mothers and fathers in 1988 indicated that men were more likely to want larger numbers of children than their partners; all women interviewed wanted no more than they had at the time of the conversation (between two and four), whereas all the fathers wanted more than they had (between one and six) (Burbank and Chisholm 1992:180). In this material we can also see a source of gender difference in ideas about ideal family size: a male bias in pivotal social arrangements and a consequent desire for sons:

> I've got a part to play in ceremony too. I've got songs, ceremonial things. Land too. If I get old, I know that I've got a son, he might take responsibility of the ceremony and the country. Somebody who will take over and my family will go on and on. Instead of just having a family, we could have just lived on with no kids, that would have been the end of [my] family line...With our first child we were really happy...and we decided to have another. Our real aim was to have a boy, but we didn't have that until we had three girls, then we had a boy, and I think we're finished. (Aboriginal man in Burbank and Chisholm 1992:183)

Circumstances of culture, history, and biology may have conspired with men against women in this regard. I have presented an example of fetal plasticity with reference to the number of cells in a kidney. A second example of human plasticity is seen in physiological systems that maintain a balance between a woman's own energy reserves and those dedicated to gestation or lactation. The label "maternal depletion syndrome" identifies a physiological state where this balance is upset. Insufficiently long birth spacing is one source of interference. Maternal depletion is thought to undermine the health of both mother and offspring; in the later case it may lead, among other things, to low birth weight (Ellison 2001:94–5; Shell-Duncan and Yung 2004).

Cole (1982) has emphasized the near-coincidence of Numbulwar's establishment as the Rose River Mission with the Commonwealth's policy of assimilation, implemented in the Northern Territory's Welfare Ordinance of 1953: "Every endeavour was made to change them from being nomads into people living settled lives in communities...They were taught health and hygiene and worthwhile trades and occupations" (15). In the mission's early years, most adult residents were required to work, though pregnant and lactating women were exempted. Together, the missionaries and their flock constructed an airstrip, sawmill, church, clinic, school, and houses (Young 1981:173). Indigenous residents were paid for their work: "No rations are issued to the people. They have to work for wages and may buy their flour and rice, etc. at the sales stores" (Montgomerie 1954 Annual Report in Cole 1982:34). Yet people were expected to obtain a substantial proportion of their food from the surrounding bush. Until 1958, supplies arrived by boat from Roper Mission only every six months. When they were low, Aboriginal residents were sent "walkabout" (Cole 1982:34, 38; Young 1981:173).

Soon, however, food became plentiful. Reviewing early mission materials, Young (1981) paints a picture of this abundance:

> When mission construction was completed, attention turned towards increasing local food production, mainly for consumption within the community. This was so successful that it became apparent that Numbulwar could provide a considerable surplus, particularly in fruit, vegetables and eggs. In 1959/60 the market garden produced 4 tons of fruit and vegetables but in 1965/66 this had increased to over 40 tons, approximately a pound per day for every[one] on the settlement... [F]or a number of years Numbulwar exported eggs for workers for the Groote Eylandt Mining Company (GEMCO). In the absence of a market, Numbulwar garden crops were distributed freely throughout the community or, on occasion, were left to rot. (174)

> In 1956 over 150 dugong, yielding about 45,000 lbs of meat, were bought by the mission from the fishermen of Numbulwar. (194)

Once the mission became a sustainable community, people ceased moving from place to place in the manner of their hunting and gathering past. By the 1970s when the outstation movement began and more people again traveled more extensively, they routinely used vehicles and motorized boats to do so.

The hunting and gathering lifestyle of groups such as the Kung, as reported by Howell (1979), is one associated with a particular pattern of fertility. This is characterized by a relatively late age of menarche, followed by a relatively prolonged period of sub-fecundity, and a completed reproductive history of four or five births spaced about four years apart by periods of lactational amenorrhea (Lancaster 1986:17–18). Cowlishaw (1981) has argued on the basis of a compilation of biological, ethnographic, and historical material that this was probably the pre-contact reproductive pattern of Indigenous Australians. She also observed the increase in fertility, the lengthening of the fertile period, and the decrease in birth spacing among women on missions and government settlements. In particular, she noted the association of this new fertility profile with changes in energy expenditure and diet.[10]

Currently, women at Numbulwar appear to lead a physically less strenuous life than they or their ancestors did in their hunting and gathering days. McArthur's (1960) observations of subsistence practices in Arnhem Land in the 1940s included a hunting and gathering group on Bickerton, an island just a few kilometers off the coast from Numbulwar with an environment similar to that of the mainland (160). McArthur remarked of the women's food quest that it was "a job which went on day after day without relief," though "they rested quite frequently and did not spend all the hours of daylight searching for or preparing food" (92). No comparable drain on women's energy expenditure appears to have arisen since settlement. With much of women's subsistence role rendered unnecessary by the availability of energy rich flour and sugar (see Altman 1984; 1987) and with the need to remain near at hand because children are at school, an institution the reader will recall was established at Numbulwar in 1953, women's daily lives have taken a decidedly sedentary turn.

It is also apparent that women have been consuming more calories than in the past. In April of 1979, Young surveyed the purchases made by Aboriginal people in Numbulwar's shop. Her survey indicated "excessive" consumption of "flour, bread and sugar" in particular and a daily caloric intake almost double that recommended. While she admits that the use of shop expenditure to provide information on nutritional intake is very rough, the accuracy of her finding is suggested by increasing amounts of obesity to be seen in men, women, and children (Young 1981:225–7).

What were the possibilities for women with bodies more receptive to pregnancies they may not have desired and that might have injured their health or that of the developing fetus? Contraceptive use would have been an option, but the mission run health service does not appear to have provided birth control methods, at least on a widespread basis, until the 1970s. An analysis of 232 live births to 73 mothers between 1925 and 1988 shows a decrease in the mean interbirth interval from over 50 months in the period 1925–1949 to 26–29 months between 1965 and 1980. By 1988, a reversal of the interbirth interval appeared, increasing to 39 months (Burbank and Chisholm 1989:89–90). This was likely due to greater access to contraception.

During this study I was able to ask a woman with a long experience of the health clinic about the availability of birth control devices:

> VKB: When the missionaries were here could women get family planning from the clinic?
>
> AW: In those days, I remember, for family planning, it never never been said. Only in traditional way that I been telling you. But in Western way family planning had not been brought out. The nurse knew and I was learning about it but we never talked to young woman or old woman because they couldn't understand. But now they know it. The nurse never said it. Later in the years, finally it came up. They can take loops. Later in the time when it started, I was interpreting, talking to the older ones. Young ones [use it] today. I had a group of women to discuss it with. Some didn't make sure they wanted it, but some did. Just the loops. They didn't have much to send out. Older ladies got loops because they had nother one coming, nother one coming. Just to have a rest.
>
> VKB: Was that in the old clinic [building] or the new clinic?
>
> AW: In the old clinic. You were in the caravan down with your abuji [kin term for FM, the year was 1978]. (AW 2003)

The extent to which women employed traditional contraceptive practices, regarded as "women's business," is unknown. According to women like this speaker, the result of these is permanent infertility.

Stress

To say that until contraception was provided, the missionaries controlled Aboriginal women's fertility is an exaggeration that nevertheless makes an important point. The literature on "social determinants of health" (e.g., Wilkinson 1996) suggests that this kind of control may have had consequences beyond those of contributing to circumstances where women bore more children than was healthy or desired.

There is much to suggest that primates, including humans, may be acutely aware of their own advantage or disadvantage vis-à-vis social rank and material wealth, though in our case cultural systems may work to diminish this awareness to some extent. We are also learning that awareness of subordination and disadvantage is an experience that is often if not always disliked by humans (e.g., Boehm 2004:279) and may be accompanied by harmful stress (Brunner and Marmot 1999; Sapolsky 2004). It is likely that negative stress would be even greater when material disadvantage and social subordination are experienced in association with an ascribed identity that has been the target of extreme violence, albeit much of this is now past. The mothers of Numbulwar whom I encountered during the study period may be the fourth or fifth generation of women whose bodies and minds have been stressed, if not by maternal depletion then by experiences of social and material disadvantage. It is becoming increasingly clear that while undernutrition may be the basis of the fetal origins of ill health and disease, this may not simply be due to what women eat. Maternal constraint, that is, the maternal capacity to nurture a fetus, may also be affected by a woman's health status, which may have begun during her own fetal origins (e.g., Adair and Prentice 2004; Barker 1994; Drake and Walker 2004; Harding 2001). In this discussion of the early days of Numbulwar, I have suggested a number of sources that may have challenged maternal capacity. These include maternal depletion and the stresses arising from relative poverty and a disadvantaged position in the social hierarchy. Sadly, these experiences are not simply history.

Chapter 4

Feeling Bad: Everyday Stress

Harmful, Threatening, and Challenging Conditions

Whitefellas visiting Numbulwar during the years of this study might, within a day or two, think they had identified a multitude of "harmful, threatening, or challenging conditions" (Lazarus 1999:36). The physical environment was one of noise and dirt. Signs of overuse and disrepair were everywhere. Walls were covered in graffiti, shade trees had been hacked down, and empty soft drink cans, cigarette butts, and other debris littered the ground. CD players, electric instruments, and homemade drums provided a soundtrack that sometimes dominated daily, and nightly, life. Dogs, often lean and sometimes diseased, appeared in packs. Vehicles constantly moved on the few roads that intersected the township, occasionally at dangerous speeds. From time to time, violence threatened; a man might stalk up to the Council building armed with spears, an axe, or a sword; a woman might broadcast verbal abuse and overturn rubbish bins as she made her way along the road bisecting the central part of town.

There were also less immediately visible, but soon obvious, indications of harmful, threatening, and challenging conditions. It was not necessary to enter the health clinic to see its constant stream of patients, men, women, and children. Even perfunctory and casual conversations with town inhabitants revealed community quarrels and family tensions over too-scarce resources. They also revealed cases of truancy, drug-induced psychoses, other forms of serious ill health, disability, and grief over the death of family members. Loudspeaker announcements from the Council office on most weekday mornings informed the listener that young people were running around at night, sometimes with weapons, breaking into the shop, office, and clinic; they broadcast the news that young people had run out of ganja and had threatened to curse the shop. From the loudspeaker one learned that sores could spread from dogs to people; that if people seriously damaged their houses they would have to pay for them; that if mothers "love" their children they would take them to the clinic, cook for them, and not smoke ganja in the house. It was from the office loudspeaker that I learned of a "body comin' "; and from the regular procession of bodies returned from the Darwin morgue, and the funerals that followed, I was reminded, should such reminding be necessary, of what was often the end consequence of these conditions.

Emotion Talk and Bad Things

I cannot proceed any further, however, without first asking, as I do repeatedly in this book, if what I as a visitor might see as stressful circumstances were experienced as such by people at Numbulwar. It is at such a moment that I recall the recent view of feelings as evolved mechanisms for responding to environmental challenges (e.g., Ribeiro et al. 20051265). Before turning to some of the emotion talk in the texts, which should allow me to address this concern, I remind myself, and the reader, of the discussion about emotions and their link to stress presented in chapter one. There are two points to keep in mind here, both relevant to my assumption of a general human inclination to name feelings arising from stress. First, people anywhere can be expected to talk about emotions more generally: they talk about feeling "good" or "bad," they describe the scenarios that accompanying feelings, and they describe physical sensations that are a part of the emotional experience. Second, words signifying anger-like, fear-like, and shame-like feelings are likely to be a part of any lexicon (Wierzbicka 1999). Luckily, just such terms as "anger," "fear," and "shame" have been linked, both theoretically and empirically, to stressful experiences (e.g., Lazarus 1999; Panksepp 1998). We cannot be surprised then to find that people at Numbulwar talk about "feeling good" and "feeling bad," describe scenarios of which feelings are a part, talk about physical sensations that accompany more cerebral experiences, and use emotion words that may be translated as "anger-like," "fear-like," and "shame-like." This content in their narratives has enabled me to learn about experiences they have that may be accompanied by activations of the "fight or flight" response and represent them here with some confidence in their psychological validity (Wallace 1961:87).

I find an exemplary starting point in Raelene's (2003) discussion of feeling bad in relation to the death of family members:

Raelene: Sometimes I feel bad inside in my life.
VKB: You feel bad, what for?
Raelene: About my family passed away.

Given that death, more than any other human experience, is likely to invoke both a fear-like and anger-like response (Bowlby 1980:85, 128–9; Durkheim 1915:439, 447; Robben 2004:2–3), I take deaths of other people, especially those whom we know and care about, as an exemplar of stressful circumstances. It is not surprising that Raelene has made a connection between death and feeling "bad." Nor, given death's prevalence at Numbulwar, is it surprising that other people speak about death, particularly about the loss of family:

I been sad to go in the airplane, go to the funeral. I been sad to go to families. When you sad, you think about that fella left you and you sit and crying and worry, think about that fella. Or they fight, make you sad, upset. When they kill [strike or kill] father, son, with spears, make you upset. Someone sick, make you feel sad or your family passed away, make you sad. (Sherry 2005)

We have here in Sherry's exegesis on the Kriol word "sad" a string of additional words and phrases that may be used to describe feeling "bad": "sit and crying," "worry," and "upset." These words expand our knowledge of the vocabulary used at Numbulwar to talk about feeling bad. In her text, Sherry also provides us with several other scenarios that increase our acquaintance with circumstances associated with bad feelings: the illness, injury, or attack on someone, especially someone who is "family." It is notable that in all the examples she provides, Sherry feels sad for the misfortune of others. This includes her feelings of sadness occasioned by other's grief, implied in her mention of seeing the "families" she would visit should she go to another community to attend a funeral.

In the texts of a third woman, the eighteen-year-old Kinsey, I find another phrase linked to the death of family members scenario, that of "don't like" when she says, "I don't like people to die" and in others' texts I find "don't like" used to label less dramatic but apparently unpleasant aspects of life at Numbulwar. Here, for example, is a comment from a much older woman, Majiwi (2004), first encountered in chapter two:

> People here, the way they use their words. They don't like the way
> they say words, they don't like, it's not normal. They sometimes don't
> respect, like young people, they don't respect older one. And their
> way, they don't pleased with, here, when they saying nasty things,
> that word when they not respecting people. Everybody feel uncom-
> fortable because he shouldn't be saying bad words. When I went to
> pick up today [a handicapped girl] at the office and a guy come in,
> somebody, saying any word. Just to be show off. Words insulting to
> hear but people not interested. I said to [a woman], "What's wrong
> with him?" "He just saying anyhow, so people can see him and he
> can show off." Yapping away that young man. Nobody been say any-
> thing. He just showing off, telling anybody. Our ways, of Aboriginal
> people, they can be nasty to each other, making up stories and try
> and make everybody to talk, asking questions about that person in
> the story, [but really] nothing to prove it. Old people can't ask him,
> they don't want to take notice of nasty story for somebody else.

Older people, such as Majiwi, don't like it when others, who often
seem to be younger people these days, use obscene language, especially in a public setting where both men and women are present.
Similarly, gossip, while frequently practiced and greatly appreciated
in private settings, to judge by the many such lively conversations
I have taken part in, has, on more than one occasion, precipitated a
fight. Words, especially "nasty" ones, that is, sexual in content, can
lead to "trouble," often of a physical and aggressive nature (Burbank
1994:51). I resume discussion of this possibility momentairly.

Sherry's (2004) discussion of infidelity adds to our knowledge
about things that people don't like:

> They having a problem, you know they have a problem with husband,
> sometime fight and jealousing. That make them feel upset. And they
> go somewhere else, maybe Darwin. Stay there. And when their hus-
> band trick them, get another woman, and they go Darwin, Katherine,
> Roper, Yirkalla, Milingimbi, they find other man, they married. They
> find new husband, old husband jealous them, they go and find their
> own. Because she having a problem, she want to find another man,
> to take care of her. They find a nice man to take care of her. Well,
> the man here they married, they go to town, they get a woman. They
> asking question, "What you do?" "Oh, your husband been tricking
> you, get one woman." And make feel upset, sad. Woman says now,
> "I don't like him now. I'll go away, find another man." You know, like
> [woman], she was having a hard time for [her husband].

The women in Sherry's account not only don't like their husbands, they are "having a hard time," they feel "upset" and "sad" due to this series of events. Adultery, or suspicions of adultery, frequently leads to jealousy and fighting and sometimes to the search for a new marital partner. When tension arises between couples, partners don't necessarily go to town or find new ones there, as in Sherry's scenario. Hence the anger and aggression associated with infidelity is enacted in the midst of people they know and who often have obligations to protect and support them though this may require acts of physical restraint if not aggression (Burbank 1994).

Returning to the paradigmatic circumstance of stress, that is, the death of others, Peg (2003), a recent widow, illustrates an experiential connection between a spouse's death and feeling "angry" when she says: "When I first lost my husband I was falling apart and angry and blaming myself that it was my fault and I was not thinking straight and I was thinking about dying too." Not only is Peg "falling apart," "blaming" herself , "not thinking straight," and "thinking about dying too," expressions I rarely if ever heard from others, she is also "angry" and this is a word often associated with more mundane occurrences. Merry provides us with two domestic scenarios that precipitate this emotion in her experience:

> I won't tell you about my family, too hard. Kids fighting, especially [two eldest sons] humbugging [bothering or fighting with her two youngest sons]. I give them hiding. That make me worried, too much. Make me sad when I growl at my kids. And after a while I sit down and after I say sorry to them. When I feel angry I use nasty word and I feel sorry I use the nasty word to my kids. [My eldest son] is too much walking around, copying other kids, stupid kids, make him want to go boil [make him angry]. He goes home, he sees young people here and goes home and humbug [my two youngest sons]. I don't know their life maybe; they do it that way. Sometimes I talk strongly, not to follow those spoiled kids. (Merry 2004)

> Don't tell me night time! One man got stereo he got, making noise all night. I can't sleep. Maybe finish up at 2:00 or 3:00. Real one what I'm saying, true story. When your uncle here, he always growl at that man to not making noise because sometime he have grog shake, because he had too much grog. [When your uncle growls], he stop, but yesterday he was making noise all night because your uncle not here. When they make the noise, I can't sleep and I get up. When he finish making the noise, when he finish, I go back to sleep, like nap, for little time because noise in the morning. And right now he's there,

listening to the tape. Sometime we tell [my husband's elder brother] to talk to him not to make noise. When [my husband] sleep and he make noise, [my husband] get up and want to growl at him but he feel sorry for him. Because he's [handicapped]. I get nervous. If you talk to [his mother] to tell him not to make noise...if she go and talk to him, he growl at [his mother] too. If you tell him to shut it off he get angry, he got two shovel spears [spears with metal spear heads] and one stick, *mabargu* [stick], at that house. (Merry 2004)

Merry also provides us both with new words for talking about bad feelings and expands our knowledge of the scenarios in which we might use some others we have already learned. She is angry when her children behave badly, "sad" and "worried" when she punishes them. She reflects on her own acts of aggression by feeling "sorry," while her husband feels sorry enough for an inconsiderate neighbor to suppress his own aggressive impulses. One of her emotion descriptors, "go boil," is, as far as I know, a neologism. It appears, nevertheless, to be a spontaneous manifestation of a widely distributed conceptual metaphor, *anger is a pressurized container*, that structures understanding of what we call anger in standard English, Chinese, Japanese, Hungarian, Wolof, and Polish (Kövecses 2005:39). "Nervous" was not a word commonly used at Numbulwar in my experience, but "hard" was, often as in "having a hard time," demonstrated in Sherry's discussion of marital infidelity provided earlier.

Finally we return to just feeling bad. Again the teenage Kinsey (2005) speaks:

> *Kinsey*: [My life] it's now bad. Because people growling at me, makem me upset. And making me worry about, like worry inside, making me think about my father mob. If people like growling at me and make me upset, that's why. Or talk about you behind your back and you don't know, that make you upset and worry and skinny.[1]
> *VKB*: What's that behind the back talk?
> *Kinsey*: Anything, like maybe talk about you for anything, or they jealous to you, you know, like girl. They talk about you for anything.
> *VKB*: Other girls been talk about you?
> *Kinsey*: Yeh.
> *VKB*: What for that behind the back talk make you think about your father?
> *Kinsey*: Maybe they talk about me and make me upset and make my father and mother upset too. They gonna talk to them too. My mother and father like me, they are going to say to them, I don't tease anybody, I don't jealous anybody, I'm just walking around myself

and be happy to my family. They talking to that girl. Like explain with them not to teasing, "Cause you might make a big problem, your mother and father might end up fighting," with my mother and father, and stab each other. They might stab each other, eh?

We learn from Kinsey's text not only more about the circumstances that are associated with feeling bad but also something of the local theory about feeling bad, principally that other people can make us feel bad. They can make us feel bad by teasing us, being jealous of us, growling at us, and talking about us behind our back. And in such circumstances our family might also start feeling bad and take steps that could lead to a fight between families in which serious injury might be done. And all of this can "make you upset and worry and skinny," that is to say, as a Westerner might, "feel stressed."

In her text, Kinsey also provides us with a label that subsumes scenarios associated with feeling bad; this label is "problem." Over the three years of this study, I asked thirteen people, twelve women, and one man one or both of the following questions: "(1) What are some bad things that can happen to people? (2) What do you think are the biggest problems for people here at Numbulwar?" Not surprisingly these questions prompted overlapping replies. All of the replies are easily subsumed under six headings that I have devised: *young and old people; loss of culture; aggression, vandalism, and delinquency; health, illness, and accidents; death and sorcery*; and the most commonly mentioned problem or bad thing, *ganja* (and sometimes alcohol). While family members may feel bad for, protect, support, and defend each other, they may also demand ganja and grog, or the money to buy it.

Ganja and Grog

The subjective, psychological effects of smoking cannabis can be compared with the pleasures of alcohol: a disconnection with the ordinary world of worries and expectation, a pronounced sense of amusement, the ability to laugh more, as well as an impaired cognitive reasoning ability. In short, we see again a drift away from abstracted logical reasoning tendencies that characterize the human mind in favour of a more emotional perspective, one focused on the immediate here and now.

—Greenfield 2000:80

People's "logical reasoning tendencies," I suspect, have led them to see, in one way or another, that the extent of their countrymen's dysfunction, disease, disability, and death presages no shining future for them. Why not attempt to eradicate this vision?

A related means of discussing the connection between a stressful social environment and drug use is provided by the self-medication hypothesis, the idea that drug use is motivated by an attempt to manage emotional distress (Khantzian 1985). While the use of this hypothesis in the psychiatric literature focuses on the co-occurrence of drug addiction and psychiatric disorders (and Numbulwar cannot be regarded as a population of the mentally ill), recent use of "stress" as a construct to understand the relationships between substance abuse and psychiatric disorders is highly relevant to my concerns. The utility of applying the stress construct to understand this relationship has been demonstrated in a variety of ways. For example, a review of recent work in the area (Brady and Sinha 2005) has found that one of the principal hormones of the stress system, corticotropin-releasing factor (CRF), contributes to anxiety, affective disorders, and addiction. Recent work has also demonstrated that among addicted individuals drug craving is increased by negative feelings and emotional stress. Most striking, though the empirical work is restricted to animal studies, is the finding that "Early life stress and chronic stress result in long-term changes in stress responses...Such changes can alter the sensitivity of the dopamine system to stress and can increase susceptibility to self-administration of substances of abuse" (1484). Returning to Numbulwar in 2003 after an absence of five years, I found ganja use, once scarcely known, well entrenched. Alcohol use appeared to be at least as pervasive, if not more so, than in previous years:

> *Carmel:* I remember back, early 2000 or 1998, in 1996, one fella, there was a suicide.[2] He hung himself, here at Numbulwar. We had a Police Aide then. He had to run there and see the man hanging and ring the cops. Family was there. The Police Aide had to ask Police if, "It's alright we cut him down and lay him down?" and Police said, "It's alright," so he cut him down and laid him down. He was family of mine; my mother was his full blood auntie. He is the only one I can remember so far. He had a drug habit, smoking ganja. But people say blackfella way forced him to do it. He thought some people were going to kill him. He did not want people to take his life, so he did it himself. It was a very sad day. I still remember him and when I do I shed tears and pray to God, when I think of him. He was my favourite cousin.

VKB: Why do you think some people here like to smoke ganja?

Carmel: Some get bored, they haven't got jobs. Some do for worriedness, like if their wife leave them or from argument with family. I know my two grandchildren are smoking ganja but when their father comes back home, he's really strict. But they don't listen to me. When daddy come home and see anything like bottle he'll make them pick up all the bottle and burn the bottle.

VKB: What's the bottle for?

Carmel: They use it for smoking ganja. Or he, their father, will go next door. [My grandaughter] gets that thing, ganja, there because I give them food and tobacco. So in turn they give my granddaughter smoke. My son goes after the youngest. The youngest one, girl, got no earhole [doesn't have sense].

VKB: How many do you think smoke ganja?

Carmel: Half of the school kids and half the middle aged and married couples.

VKB: How young do they start smoking?

Carmel: I would say about fourteen years old because that's how old my granddaughter is. On Groote it's about twelve or eleven.

VKB: Are there people here who drink alcohol?

Carmel: They go out of the community to drink. Only one, lazy one, get that home brew [material for making alcoholic drink] from general store on Groote. They charge $25 a bottle of home brew to make money. Here they have to pay $50 a bag for ganja. In town it's $25 a bag, in Darwin, Gove. At Batchelor [College], I was on a course there. It was getting dark, I didn't want to walk by myself so I said, "I'll have to walk with you," to some other students there. In the village they stopped and this woman lifted up her shirt and she asked, "What do you want? This one $50, this one $25," buying at Bachelor. They bring back the home brew in a boat, but nothing now, because of the coppers [whose visit to Numbulwar was due to an act of violence]. They get individual bottles, coke bottles and they fill it up with home brew and sell it for $25. One [Aboriginal] person made one grand. Like a jerry can of home brew selling, I don't know maybe for $500. He had six jerry cans full of brew, made $3000. And one fella was selling ganja, made $2600, in a week he made $1000 and another week he made another $1000. At midnight they get money from family and go to his house and buy the ganja. He is an [Aboriginal person] and he's smoking too.

VKB: Do you think there is anything good about ganja?

Carmel: I don't think so. It just make them madder and madder. Some people who smoke are losing weight, shrinking up, that dress they are wearing is too big. Some people, I'm thinking here of my grandson, he put a rag around his pants to keep his trousers up. My granddaughter is losing weight. I don't know if it's because she is getting older or the smoking is eating away her body. These are the two main things. (2003)

Not everyone at Numbulwar would have agreed with Carmel's answer to my last question. Ganja, some said, makes people happy, productive, and nonaggressive:

They reckon it good for their health, make you quiet, you can't fight after when you finish that smoke. If you smoke straight all right, but if you mix it up with tobacco, big problem when you mix it up with Log Cabin [tobacco]. (Lily 2003)

Sometime [young people] get bored. When really bored they go fishing and especially [hand sign for smoking ganja].[3] When they have that thing, make them happy. They do working, gardening, walk about, sleep. But people don't smoke that thing, they get bored. (Merry and Sherry 2004)

It was illegal to have alcoholic beverages at Numbulwar without a special permit and to my knowledge no Aboriginal person at Numbulwar has ever received one. Instead, as Carmel observes in the quote earlier, people left the community to drink, an activity referred to as "touristing."[4] Alternatively, or following a trip to town, people might attempt to smuggle grog into Numbulwar:

Some men when they go out with the vehicle, go to buy some grog with the vehicle and buy some at Katherine or Mataranka, buy some grog and come back and drinking at home and making mess and fighting, breaking houses, chase wife and kids. Some people see man, he's acting stupid, and ring cops and cops come and ask him, "What for you chasing wife and kids, breaking the new houses?" And cops tell him, "Don't touch [go near] Katherine or Mataranka," and write down the number plate of vehicle. And if they see him go past, they gonna pull him over and tell him to come out and put him in the police station and tell the man not to get the vehicle back. Like your *baba* [father], [woman's name] husband. They found that truck with lots of grog and they get that truck and put it in the police station and he's not gonna get it back now. Maybe he got money, maybe, I don't know how much, he gotta pay for vehicle to get it back. Because they was waving [gesturing] him not to go to Mataranka and Katherine, they was waving, but he didn't listen. Every Friday when they get

their pay, [woman's name] and his husband go now, buy some grog.
Because some people, they lose that vehicle. (Sherry 2005)

Agar (2003) has suggested that, along with population level factors,
we need to "consider the subjective effect" of drugs when trying to
understand epidemics of substance abuse (27). It may be no accident
that alcohol, ganja, and petrol (which is a solvent) appear to be the
drugs of choice in many remote, and not so remote, Indigenous communities (e.g., Brady 1992; Hunter 1993; Sansom 1980). According
to the psychopharmacologist Greenfield (2000), "the net effect [of
cannabis] on synaptic transmission is...similar to alcohol and sol-
vents" (80); all enable the disconnection of meaning and experience.
Thus, the perception that ganja can replace both alcohol and petrol sniffing is not surprising. Nor, given the local observation that
ganja makes people "quiet," is it surprising that at least some think
the substitution of ganja for drinking and sniffing a good thing.
Here these speakers from Numbulwar might be seen to agree with
Bourgois (2003) when he says that "individuals sometimes destroy
their lives through chronic marijuana abuse, but compared to other
drugs...marijuana is the least-of-all-evils from a social pharmaco-
logical perspective" (36). Everyone at Numbulwar has seen, if not
experienced first hand, the devastating permanent physiological
effects of sniffing petrol. All have at least witnessed repeated acts of
alcohol-precipitated violence (Burbank 1994):

> That's the main problem that's been happening in 1999, still coming
> up. I've been talking to young boys who been with ganja, "What if
> you stop this drug, what if we stop this drug coming in?" They say,
> "We go back to petrol sniffing," some of the boys said to me. So
> Council have to be aware of what might happen if we stop marijuana.
> Maybe sneak in grog or start selling home brew. That was happening
> before. We had really big problem with home brew. Police came and
> spoke with the people doing home brew. (Sawyer 2003)

In November of 2005 I was told that the police had come to
Numbulwar and had visited a household selling ganja:

> Police came last night. One fat one, one with a long mustache. The
> fat one went to the back, the mustache one went to the front door.
> And knocked and they thought maybe it was somebody wants to buy
> ganja, but it was police. And they said maybe, "Come in." They was
> playing cards at the kitchen. And they asked them for [man's name].
> He was lying down because he has flu. They found him and lots of

ganja and money and they put it in the bag and took him back to Ngukurr to jail. "Somebody rang them up," in reply to my question, "How did they know to go there?" They told them, "Somebody rang us up, but we can't tell you who." They keep it secret...Q: What for would somebody ring up? A: Maybe they asked them for one free one ganja. And when they wouldn't give them any they rang them up. They dob them in. (2005:V:76–7)

About two weeks later, in early December 2005, I observed one young man and one boy who appeared to be sniffing petrol, though throughout most of the field study people had been saying "nobody sniffing":

[Woman] around 4:00 PM at door. Comes in. Sits by window. Note [teenage girl already present] has been watching activity on beach and road during visit commenting on who is doing what...Now [woman] also observing. Says somebody sniffing petrol there, "You look, by the coconut tree, one side." I can see, now that it's pointed out to me, that someone is by the coconut tree. He's got a jerry can. He's hiding it in the bushes, by the old basketball court. He returns to jerry can, probably fills up tin and holds to face. Tall, slender, dressed in yellow and black, appears to be doing almost a dance or mime, arms extended, perhaps in conversation with invisible person, graceful. [I say], "Maybe we should tell somebody." Neither [second teenage girl] nor [first teenage girl] say anything. [Woman] indicates no, "His family don't like him now, he's cranky." [Second teenager] says, "He's going to start everybody now." And a few minutes later we see two smaller and younger looking boys approach him. One takes the sniffing can and appears to sniff briefly. Both then leave. [Second teenager] says, "No money for ganja, so they are sniffing." V: Where did they get petrol? Nobody should have petrol here. Collective answer: From [building] contractors. [Second teenager]: They sniffing Avgas. V: Can they sniff Avgas?' [Woman]: "They gonna damage their brain." Petrol sniffer is [man in mind-twenties]. His mother died, his stepmother "don't look after" him. (2005:VI:34–5)

The following day, another woman remarked, "Lots of girls and boys, school girls, young boys sniffing, because they desperate because nobody selling ganja these days." And one of the teenage observers of the previous day added, "I told you he was starting everybody" (2005:VI:43, 44).

Although some people indicate they see ganja as an improvement on alcohol and petrol, without some of their negative effects, it is also seen to have harmful social consequences:

Peg: The biggest problem is the ganja, when they smoke. I fear that young people, like ten years old, will get into it. And alcohol. When someone brings in alcohol and get into a fight, because alcohol makes you big talk and swearing. They fight with their family, with their wives. And other thing, they gonna lose their culture if they keep smoking ganja.

VKB: Why if they keep smoking ganja will they lose their culture?

Peg: I think some of the clans, they don't get up and enjoy ceremony sometime. Only the people I see, some faces like my tribe [clan], just only us. Some [clan name] don't join in with us. I want them to...keep up what they have been taught by their elders. And if elders die, all the things go with them. There will be no one else to teach us. Like in the future our grandchildren won't learn anything, and grandchildren's children. I think ganja and alcohol is the main problem. (Peg 2003)

While drinking alcohol is associated with aggression and smoking ganja with being quiet, violence is anticipated when the desire to smoke ganja is frustrated:

Some people looking for money and if no money they look for fight. They growl at them wife and tell them to go look for marijuana. It's hard. And they bash them wife and go to hospital and ring some cops. Like two weeks ago [man's name] tell [his wife] to go looking for marijuana, and to go and ask anybody. He told her, when she didn't get any, "Don't sleep here, go away, go sleep outside." It make them angry when they can't find ganja, *makem allabut wild* [making them wild]. When they smoke the ganja they sit down quiet. You can't tell *allabut*, "Leave ganja." If you tell them they can't listen to you because that thing making them good, to stop fighting, not walk around, they stay home, doing cooking, gardening and cleaning. If they can't get it, they angry, they go off. (Sherry 2003)

Adults and children have experienced the physical wrath of someone, usually a man, intoxicated from drinking or "desperate for ganja"; and, of course, both alcohol and ganja take money away from food, clothing, and other necessities.

Other Bad Things

Although I created the categories for the brief summary of bad things, it is both easy and important to see the interrelationship of their content in people's experience, their "complex and dynamic links" in people's lives. As well as ganja and grog, the aspects of life summarized by *young and old people; loss of culture; aggression, vandalism, and delinquency; health, illness and accidents; and death and sorcery* are interwoven in stressful experiences for people at Numbulwar. I begin with a look at Majiwi's (2003) answer to the question about the biggest problems for people there:

> Biggest problem is, what I think…Smoking of marijuana is a new style for young people, and even middle ages. Smoking and sometime bringing liquor in. People get drunk, like getting into drugs. Otherwise, if that couldn't have been here, could be a peaceful and happy place. Elder people not happy losing culture, but young people are interested in *wunubal* [public clan songs and accompanying dances] and traditional ways of teaching young ones. Young people are really much interested but only a few elders are teaching them. I've seen young ones really interested in the traditional ways. And then trouble comes, distressing whole of the town. Some of the people taking drugs don't care. But people with respect want to see changes and can live together. The main problem is bringing stuff in. Some people live in the bush. Young ones, women going out fishing, elder men go out in the boat. It's their life, they can get along, they can teach the young. Some young ones sitting around doing nothing, start big problem, family to family…Problem is, the family groups really worried about them. Worried that people don't take that sort of drugs, make sure they are happy enough and don't take it. Family group a bit distressed about that. That's the only thing I can think of because I see my, a lot of young ones, even maybe young up to 20 and 19, like that age, they still not on the way they should be.

Majiwi is saying that were it not for imported alcohol and drugs, Numbulwar "could be a peaceful and happy place." Young people are the principal users, especially of marijuana, and this worries their families who think they take drugs because they are not "happy." "Young ones" end up "doing nothing" and "start big problem" between families when their drug use and idleness lead them to make-trouble, that is, fight, steal, vandalize property, or otherwise misbehave. Older people are "not happy" about "losing culture," by which Majiwi means the realm of the sacred, the Dreaming or Law, and its public manifestations in dance and song. She displays some indecision about whether this loss is due to disinterest on the part of the young or the disinclination to teach the young on the part of the old. On past fieldtrips, I have been told that older people, men in particular, have not been willing to pass on sacred knowledge to a younger generation seen as unworthy of receiving it, a generation who are not "on the way they should be." The teachers are particularly likely to live on a "homeland" (outstation), practicing hunting, fishing, and gathering to some extent, for at least a part of the year. By trouble Majiwi appears to be thinking of a recent tragic death linked to drugs, discussed further later, but not, perhaps, as a specific case so much as a prototype of traumatic events more generally. "People taking drugs don't care" even about a tragic event. People "with respect," a reference to people who would probably fit into my "9–5 crowd" (see preface), do care. They "want to see changes"—they would like to see alcohol and drugs disappear—that would make it easier to avoid the kinds of events, trouble, that harm people and relationships.

A second example is provided by Merry's (2004) response to the question about bad things that can happen to people:

> Like bad way, bad way here when people pass away, people pass away, nother people come from nother country, ask why that man been die. Like Aboriginal way they *doit* [Kriol for "do it," "do something"]. That man die, like family, relationships, they get angry, wild and having over and over meeting, asking questions of all the men, why the man been die, what sort of problem or trouble. If people find out, been somebody [who used sorcery], they have meeting; meeting over and they have fight now. Because not much old people we got here for showing children for future, for ceremony. Look like children got no future here because they killing all the old people. And old people not showing culture, sacred site. Nobody here now. Especially elders, old people.

Here Merry talks about death and its links to sorcery. When people die, family members want to know why they died. In particular, they want to know if a "man" has been murdered and what kind of misdeed, "problem or trouble,"[5] provoked the attack. When sorcery is the suspected cause of death, people are not simply sad, they are "angry" and "wild." Close family discuss the case over and over and those accused of sorcery, other men, may be attacked. Sorcery is a bad thing. The death of old people has ramifications beyond the loss of a family member. Old people, who have amassed cultural knowledge over many years, are being killed by sorcery and the children they might otherwise teach will not be able to learn about their traditions. Without old people, there is "nobody here now," Aboriginal knowledge is lost.

In Majiwi's text, drugs and alcohol are directly linked to trouble and "big problem family to family," that is, hostility and aggression, and to culture loss. In Merry's text, death is linked with "problem" or "trouble", that is, misbehavior and sorcery, and with culture loss.

Reference to each of these texts enables us to read both of them
with greater understanding. We can understand that because "old
people" are being killed off "Aboriginal way," that is, with sorcery,
there is "no future," not enough teaching in "traditional ways" to
young people, who consequently are "not on the way they should
be," bringing drugs and trouble "family to family" and to "whole
of the town." Critically, neither Majiwi nor Merry is speaking simply in the abstract. Remarks Merry (2004) made moments after she
provided the text here reveal this clearly:

> *Merry*: Going to outstation and show kids whose country this is.
> That's the good life.
> *VKB*: But people aren't living on outstations, they stay here.
> *Merry*: They afraid of people killing each other.
> *VKB*: People killing each other?
> *Merry*: Black magic. Scared of black magic [sorcery], especially
> because no old people here, only young people.[6] Some people got
> no good life; maybe they scared, because of that problem, that man
> that died at [country name]. They have to stay here now. People
> stay here and enjoy themself here, not to outstation.

In this comment Merry is referring to a death that occurred early in
2003 that people continued to talk about throughout the fieldwork
period. People were staying away from the outstations because they
were afraid that they might become a target of "black magic."

Another respondent to my question about bad things also refers
to this incident of premature death:

> People feel sick and die, especially young people, sudden deaths.
> Some sorcery...like in the case of [the man who died], your *gagu*
> [kin term]. He was out with other people...When they die at young
> age, people talk it over and over, "What's the cause?" That's the
> Indigenous way. But Western way they say he died of pneumonia.
> Indigenous have more questions. Elders sit over and family members
> talk it over, have a big meeting. Only men, *walya walya* [men], not
> women, at the meeting. Saying things, different members, they didn't
> break up in a fight, just talking. If there is a car accident, "Oh, some-
> body must have been involved to cause that person to get in the acci-
> dent," like a cattle or bullock in the road to cause that. Sometimes
> when the hunting trip come, two of us going, if you disappear from
> me, you might be chasing kangaroo, and you go around and can't
> meet up with me or if we meet up later, they think I took you out
> to murder you, make it possible that somebody could murder you.
> (Zamia 2004)

Black Magic

The various accounts surrounding aspects of the death to which Majiwi, Merry, and Zamia have referred allow us to see the experiential grounds of their texts and better understand perceived connections between the various kinds of bad things and problems. The deceased, a man just approaching his forties, accompanied two other men from two other clans on a trip, either for the purpose of selling or buying ganja at a place somewhere to the northeast of Numbulwar. During the trip, according to the various accounts, the man either left the vehicle, became lost and died of dehydration and exposure, or was the victim of sorcery and/or a more direct violent physical assault. People at Numbulwar not being notified of the man's disappearance, or being notified but delaying to act, a search party did not go out until it was too late. The man's travel companions were regarded as prime suspects by many, though not by their close family members or the police, and neither resided at Numbulwar during the fieldwork period. A series of meetings was held at Numbulwar over the years, but the death continued to be a source of distress, particularly for the man's parents and other close kinsmen.

Majiwi's response to the question about bad things happening captures the bad feelings that can surround a premature and mysterious death and lead to further trouble, and stress, in the community:

> A young lady or young man, might all of a sudden pass away... Family might say someone must have done it. Black magic. The body is taken away by police. Something must have caused that death and police do the autopsy and write back and let family know. The letter is only for family. But Indigenous people in family really concerned that someone done it. But nothing, they don't understand it. Many Indigenous people been like that, they don't understand it... start arguing, family to family, start arguing every time, even through they got that story from the doctor. Maybe later they understand. They get angry, talking angry word, using insulting words. Maybe take a long time to get sorted out. Until they come to know, more story coming up from another family [talk and questioning continues between families]. Long time, and then they forget. (Majiwi 2004)

Feeling Bad

As I listen to the women who have been speaking in this chapter, my understanding of their daily lives becomes more informed by their

willingness to share ordinary but difficult experiences with me. Some
of my first impressions about stress are on the mark. Noise, aggression, ill health, death, and substance abuse are seen as problems;
I hear from these speakers that these aspects of their environment
make them, and other people, feel bad. At the same time, however,
I also see that facets of these experiences of harmful, threatening,
and challenging conditions are culturally specific. They include
dimensions outsiders would not, at least initially, expect. While we
are not surprised to hear that the death of kin is stressful for many,
unless we have prior knowledge of Australian Aboriginal belief systems, we would neither anticipate nor understand how substantially
ideas about black magic contribute to the distress accompanying
such deaths. Without knowledge of local acts, events, and consequences and how local Aboriginal people interpret these, we would
not understand how ideas about ganja use and "losing culture" are
connected to losses occasioned by death. Nor would we understand
how thoughts about family and violence, and associated feelings,
such as "angry" and "worry," reverberate in this experience.

We have already learned from Kinsey *that other people can make
us feel bad*. If we apply what we have learned of this local theory to
the quintessentially stressful condition, death of kin, we can further
explicate at least some of the interconnections of this content. The
local theory of feeling bad can be used as a template for the local
understanding of death, a linguistic analogue to what, working at
a cognitive level, we might identify as a schema for feeling bad. In
this extension or projection of the theory of feeling bad to help us
understand death, *other people can make us feel bad* becomes *other
people can make us die*.[7] They make us feel bad by being jealous,
growling, and talking behind our back. They make us die by direct-
ing black magic at us. When we feel bad our family feels bad too.
When we die our family feels bad. When our family feels bad like
this they take actions that may lead to physical aggression.

Importantly, family may occupy either a supportive or threatening
role in this scheme of things. Family not only identify with and respond
to our bad feelings, but may sometimes be the other people who make
us feel bad. Family don't just harass us for money and drugs:

> They were blaming his brother, saying he sold him because he put
> a curse and so they wouldn't get him. He sold his younger brother.
> Stories get back to family and they feel bad. They said men came in
> boats from Groote to kill him and paid someone from Numbulwar
> to help them. (2004:I:6)

The person speaking here is saying that a man who used the strategy of cursing, perhaps inappropriately, "cursing things over and over," consequently feared he might become the target of black magic himself and therefore was willing to act in concert with others who wished to harm his brother. Thus *other people who can make us feel bad and make us dead* becomes *family who can make us feel bad and make us dead*. And all of this can "make you upset and worry and skinny"; all of this is stressful. Talk about black magic is a verbal instantiation of a "social logic" (McKnight 2005:xxviii), the social logic for "feeling bad."

The parallels between this social logic or theory of feeling bad/death and what Reid (1983) has called the "Yolngu sociomedical theory" are, of course, immediately apparent to those familiar with her ethnography, *Sorcerers and Healing Spirits*. In her prescient analysis, Reid observes that "sorcery is an extremely powerful concept, explaining as it does both how and why an illness or death occurs" (113). It provides "a sense of control" (92) and "a coping strategy at times of extreme psychological or social stress" (114). She also observes that the sociomedical theory persists regardless of extensive social change because it is "devastatingly true." Yolngu people have learned from experience "that vulnerability and trouble lead to sickness and death" (153). Discussing a string of recent deaths at Numbulwar, a visiting whitefella doctor exclaimed, "I could almost begin to believe in black magic myself." The conditions of everyday existence in this remote community would seem almost to require a theory like that of black magic.[8]

It is not yet clear, however, why family may be the *other people who make us dead*. It seems intuitive when addressing this question to turn to experiences within the kindred. My choice, however, is more theory driven than it may first appear. When I focus on a theory such as *family can make us dead*, I recognize this as a particular instantiation of the model or schema of self with others that emerges, or so it is postulated, from early attachment experiences (Bowlby 1969). Though modified throughout life, at the core of this schema we find feelings labeled by attachment theorists as "separation anxiety" and "felt security," feelings that, Panksepp (1998) argues, though not identical experiences across species, are essential to the survival of all mammals.[9] In the ideal attachment experience (but see Chisholm 1993), children feeling separation anxiety seek contact with their primary caretaker who responds in such a way that feelings of anxiety turn into feelings of security. However, even the most conscientious of caretakers has bad moments, if not bad days, and an attachment cycle reunion may include parental acts, or circumstances, such that the child's feelings of anxiety are not banished or not entirely banished and thus accompany and complicate the feelings of security (Chisholm 1999). Thus the core schema of self with others is not simply *other people can make us feel good*, but the more complex *other people can make us feel good and/or bad*. As it seems highly probable that this schema is shared by the vast majority of humans who have ever lived, I need more than ideas about general models of self with other/s to understand why family may be the *other people who can make us dead* at Numbulwar.

Family Good and Bad

Hence I turn to some of the experiences of family in this community. Participant observation over the years reveals a picture of child socialization that resembles those of other remote communities (e.g., Berndt 1978; Hamilton 1981). Aboriginal people at Numbulwar, for the most part, continue to practice a highly responsive form of early child-care that appears to be in harmony with the sustaining role that family plays in people's lives. In early years, children are kept close at hand, often in a mother's arms or at her breast, though from the 1990s onward, a growing use of prams has meant that many infants are less often in direct body contact with others. In the local environment this style makes sense. As the reader might by now intuit, there are numerous hazards, both physical and social, that challenge any carer's ability to raise a healthy child. Inadequate housing, poor sanitation, rapid fluctuation of food supply, a large domestic dog population, and the local practices of expressing anger in physical fights or by driving vehicles at considerable speed through the community streets are some challenges to which any carer must respond (Burbank and Chisholm 1992:179). The propinquity that caretakers, mothers especially, maintain with children up to the age of four or five is undoubtedly a strategy for minimizing the potential harm of these threats to children's well-being. Even school is not allowed to interfere with caretaker-child contact. Attendance at the Infants Class might begin at age three, but mothers usually attend with their children. Caretakers are also welcome to accompany their children in the Preschool Class held for four-year-olds.

Generally, mothers are quick to respond—feeding, carrying, comforting, and protecting children—as soon as a child's need is seen or expressed. Usually, young children are prevented from crying, for example, by being given what they ask for or seem to want. They are, at the same time, granted, at least symbolically, a notable degree of autonomy and so are asked, as a matter of course, about their desires to be with specific people, go to specific places, or engage in specific activities (Burbank 2006; Burbank and Chisholm 1992; see also Cowlishaw 1982; Hamilton 1981; Myers 1986:110).

The idea that secure feelings result from such early experiences would not, I think, be challenged by attachment theorists (e.g., Bretherton 1985). For example, I present what I see as a manifestation of this security in an observation I made in 2004, though the child was in a situation that seemed, if only momentarily, threatening:

> A few minutes later [an adolescent child-minder] comes out of the office holding [a little girl], about one year in age, in her arms. She stands in the passage with the baby on her hip looking toward the clinic for several minutes. The baby gazes at [a white woman] and smiles. A few minutes later [a teenage girl] comes into the passage, moves quickly over to the child-minder, claps her hands on the baby's cheeks and gives her a kiss somewhere in the middle of her face. Her movement is abrupt and fast. As she moves away from the baby she pinches its nose. The baby doesn't do anything that I can see. No flinch, cry, whimper. She does push her face down onto the breast of the carer who continues to hold but otherwise ignores the baby. (2004:VIII:89)[10]

Yet, neither childhood nor family life more generally is one of unmitigated good. Along with Chisholm (Burbank and Chisholm 1989), I have suggested that increasing family size and decreasing birth spacing have undermined mothers' ability to practice according to the ideals of this style of child care, one associated with hunter-gatherers more generally and in the earlier literature referred to as a "nurturant-indulgent" form (Burbank and Chisholm 1992). As this is a highly nurturing and responsive one, the competing needs and demands of other children necessarily interfere with it to some degree, leading to experiences that caretakers may find stressful insofar as they find themselves falling short of their own expectations. Children too would find their expectations being violated in these circumstances. Significantly, this kind of experience may add to children's *other people can make us feel bad* component of the self with others schema, either because a caretaker is not responding to the child or because another child is competing with them, sometimes aggressively.

Family life, as students of its Western forms have learned in recent decades, is not simply one of support and succor. Closer to my subject matter, Senior (2003) has proposed that families at Ngukurr are "a source of stress as well as comfort" (138). In chapter three, I suggested that people at Numbulwar experienced their relative poverty and that these experiences are a source of harmful stress. In a scenario that bears considerable resemblance to that of the Western Arrente painted by Austin-Broos (2003), I propose that such experiences are exacerbated by the interaction of two factors. One of these is the practice of demand sharing. Peterson (1993) has argued, on the basis of extensive ethnographic evidence, that demand sharing, widespread throughout Indigenous Australia and hunter-gatherer society more generally, is "deeply embedded" in Aboriginal life. On the basis of his own experience in Arnhem Land, and that of anthropologists working elsewhere in Indigenous Australia (e.g., Myers 1988; Sansom 1988), he casts demand sharing as a mechanism for the production and maintenance of relatedness (870). By asking someone for something, one may be attempting to obtain a desired good, but of greater affective and social importance, one is attempting to produce, maintain, or test a relationship, as when one of TeeJay's teenage "sisters" said to me, "If you love me, give me those apricots" (2003:VIII:89).

The second factor in this volatile mix is the sheer variety and amount of stuff that people at Numbulwar may, at least in theory, obtain (see also Austin-Broos 2003:125). Peterson (1993) has suggested that "wealth differentials, disruption, poverty or the entrenching of social inequality...may have intensified the practice" of demand sharing (870), a suggestion that I think captures the state of affairs I have observed at Numbulwar. Not only did people demand food, tobacco, drugs, money, and clothing from their kin, they demanded things such as CDs, DVDs and CDs, and DVD players, or at least their use, rides in vehicles, co-signed loans so that new vehicles could be purchased and money for flights to or from Numbulwar. Among the Arrente, women lock their refrigerators (Austin-Broos 2003:126). At Numbulwar, people stayed home to guard their video or CD collection. Catalogues, of almost any kind, were favorite reading material; many people had televisions, and all had access to television viewing, including the viewing of advertisements. The shop stocks major appliances such as refrigerators and washing machines. People may order items such as pool tables and television sets from town. Along with the new houses people occupy seems to come a desire for things like "big pillows" and "curtains" and pictures to hang on the wall.

If we assume that demands arise not only from need, but from a form of social calculus,[11] that *someone who is just like me has more than I have*, we can see the ever increasing array of objects to be possessed and associated desires to possess them generating stress above and beyond that which might accompany the acquisition of a desired object. Just as Altman and Peterson (1988) noted of Gunwinggu people on Momega's outstation, large consumer items, once purchased, however the means of doing so, are seen as legitimate objects to demand (82–3). Some may be shared in situ, as family might gather in the house that contains the TV and DVD player or washing machine. Yet, it appears that money, long a desired object, is becoming even more important. In the following text, whether money is shared or not appears to drive at least some relationships, even beyond their reciprocal aspects:

> If you winning at the card and family ask you for $20, they make you lose all the money, make you angry inside and you growling "You make me lose the money, we need the money to buy something at the shop" ... Yeah, look [speaker's kinswoman]. She like playing cards. She can't give up. She play every day. She go to [my father] and she asking for money for card. She like money, to win money, to buy baby clothes for her baby. When she get money, if she win money, she's gonna gave you back money. But family she's not gonna gave back money. Only to me, she like me. You know why? Because I was kind to her when we was young. But other mob people if they ask, she can't give. Only me and [my father]. Especially she don't give her auntie, [name] and [name] and [name]. Only she give her father and [father's brother] and [another father's brother]. She don't give auntie and father [another of father's brothers]. She don't like them because her auntie and father [name] don't give her money when they got money. Only [father's brother, her father] and [her mother] and she don't go them place, only come to [father's brother] and [my father's] house. (Kinsey 2005)

Kinsey tells us here about one of her "family"; a major determinant of this young woman's feelings about her kin is whether or not people share money with her. She avoids some family members, even though they are "close," neglects to pay them back, and refuses their requests.

In the following comment from two teenage girls, money is cast as a person in a relationship, indicating perhaps its emotional importance, at least in some circumstances: "[A man] and [a woman] have phones 'because they pay quick.' Not [another woman] and [another

man], 'because they love money,' they 'can't let go' " (2003:IX:63).
The following account from my field notes suggests the painful feelings that may accompany rejection of a request for money, arising
in large part, I think, because it is not only the request that was
being denied but also the relationship to the person (see also Myers
1986:115):

> [Woman] tells me [her sister] got her "bonus money today, $3000."[12]
> And she gave $200 to [her eldest brother] and she gave to [her eldest
> sister and her daughter] and to her [mother's sister's daughter and her
> daughter and son]. When [speaker] asked her for $50 for [her son]
> to buy a toy car from the shop, she said she didn't have any money.
> "She made me upset. When I asked her she got angry and made me
> shame." Q: "Why didn't she give you something?" A: "She's greedy,
> she's going selfish now. She didn't give me or [a third sister]." Asks if
> I have [her mother's] number in town. She's going to call and tell her
> that [her sister] didn't give anything [to the third sister]. "She always
> come to me asking me for sugar, for Rinso [laundry soap]. I told
> her, 'Don't give that $50 to me. If you give me $50, I'll burn it with
> a lighter.' She gave it to [my husband]. I told her not to come to my
> house. She made me feel upset." (2004:X:68)

Given that family is experienced as the primary and near-exclusive
source of support, as I believe it is, even momentary and seemingly
minor repudiations of relatedness, such as this, may be threatening. In this example, a woman is denied money for her child, but of
greater significance, she is not treated as other siblings are treated;
she is shamed and set apart. In retaliation, one that indicates how
"shame" and "upset" feel, she sets herself apart, at least from this
sister, by refusing the, eventually, proffered bill and telling her sister
to keep away from her. In chapter six, readers will find this response
to be in accord with a kind of family morality where relatedness is
understood in terms of "reciprocity and its negative forms of revenge
and retribution" (Lakoff and Johnson 1999:293–8). This woman,
now herself the mother of several children, also at least contemplates
calling her own mother to report her sister's behavior, though not that
directed against her but against a third sister who was also excluded
from the distribution of cash. We might wonder if even thinking
about making this call works against painful feelings insofar as it
evokes an early schema of self with others focused on a mother who
nourishes and protects, sometimes via an enabled retribution.

At the same time that relationships may be denied or invalidated,
at least briefly, by not sharing money, family not having money may

be grounds for acting less related, at least for some people: "I don't like staying with other people, [at my uncles']. They don't work, they don't have any money. I am the only one. I want a house just for myself and my two kids" (2005:P:15). Firsthand experiences of *family making me feel bad* were plentiful at Numbulwar. It is not much of a stretch for people with such experiences to also know that *family can make me dead*. While there is much more to consider about the psychological origins and functions of sorcery beliefs, I do not plan to pursue this here. Instead, I suggest that while family relationships and all they entail are a critical source of resilience, they can also be a major source of stress at Numbulwar in ways that outsiders might not anticipate.

Chapter 5

Identity

Concepts of "Self" and "Identity"

There is much to suggest that our feelings about ourselves are implicated in our health (e.g., Demakakos et al. 2008; Dressler 1991a:618–19; Taylor and Stanton 2007:379–81, 384). Or, to rephrase this in the specific terms of my argument, I anticipate that people's identity contents, depending on the nature of their subsequent experiences, may ameliorate or exacerbate the extent to which stress has harmful effects on their minds and bodies.

The concept of identity is useful here in two ways. First, it rests on an assumed relationship between individual experience and the sociocultural context of that experience, thus providing a framework consonant with my ecological approach to stress and health. Second, its use highlights internalization, that is, the idea that we learn about ourselves from others, often in emotionally charged ways, and become, to some extent, what we have learned we are. In so becoming, we act as we have learned someone like us acts and see ourselves as someone who would act that way. The concept of identity, however, also invites confusion. As in the case with so many anthropological concepts, various usages of "identity" are accompanied by diverse and sometimes incompatible models of the person (Linger 2005:160–2). Linger helps us approach, if not assimilate, this vast and unwieldy literature with a rough categorization of anthropological efforts into two camps: "the *representational* (or *public*) and *experiential* (or *personal*)" (148); the former perspective casts identity as "symbolic discursive," the latter as "mental stuff."[1] Much of the anthropological work on identity in Indigenous Australia falls into the former category.

A review of the literature on Aboriginal identity provided by M. Tonkinson (1990) distinguishes two distinct approaches of the "symbolic discursive" kind. The first of these focuses on public identities and social collectives defined largely in terms of language, kinship, and country (e.g., Austin-Broos 2009; Berndt 1977; Birdsall 1988; Merlan 2006; Trigger 1992). The second focuses on questions of just who is to be included in or excluded from a nationwide category of "Aboriginal," or more broadly, to also count Torres Strait Islanders, "Indigenous" Australians (e.g., Langton 1993; Paradies 2006). While "the personal" is often drawn upon in these latter discussions, they nevertheless continue to "treat identity as an overwhelmingly extrapersonal phenomenon" (Linger 2005:151). In contrast, Cowlishaw's (2004) ethnography of blackfella/whitefella interactions in the New South Wales town of Bourke moves identity into the "experiential" and "personal" realm when she assumes that "the intimate psychology of specific Aboriginal individuals and their interpersonal social intercourse bears a systematic relationship to a national persona, a 'social identity,'" and focuses on "the discursive identifying and reproducing of practices of identity" (8,9–10). Others, also taking a more person-centered approach, include those who see Indigenous identities as constructed through performance (e.g., McCullough 2008), art (e.g., Riphagen 2008), story (e.g., Beckett 1996), and experiences of the paranormal (Cox 2009). My effort may be placed alongside these though it differs from them in the extent to which I attempt to deal with "mental stuff," that is, with posited cognitive correlates of experiences of identity, and of self.

In Linger's discussion of the various anthropological approaches to identity, we find the term "self" used in such a way that at times the distinctions between its meaning and that of identity seem somewhat blurred. This is, I think, a good way to work with these concepts. Observing that scholars who write about self rarely include ideas about identity in their discussions and vice versa, Sökefeld (1999) proposes a model where self is given analytic priority; it is conceptualized as the agent that puts into play a given identity at a given moment.[2] This formulation of self as identity manager parallels what D'Andrade (1995) has identified as the "real self" schema in Moffatt's (n.d.) analysis of American college students' beliefs about a "true friend":

> The real self...is an internal place, where what happens is natural, unique, and *the center of human agency*...the real self is naturally spontaneous, unlike the social self, which consist of the roles and masks one has to wear in the "real world." The social self must be controlled, orderly, and on stage. (D'Andrade 1995:131; my emphasis)

It is the real self that controls the social self in this schema. It is the real self that dresses in the "roles and masks" to present a "controlled, orderly" persona while "on stage." In being conceived of so doing, the real self, or the managerial self, is cast as a "homunculus," "the idea that our mental life is controlled by an inner being who observes the world and controls our behaviour." This, Elman et al. (1996) tell us, is "one of the banes of cognitive science," "lurking in disguise in many theories" (85). Their concern, of course, is not so much that the homunculus lurks, but rather that it leads to a distorted view of mind and action. They offer in its stead a view of action as emergent, arising from the parallel activity of multiple brain/mind systems.

In accord with this latter approach, I follow Quinn (2006) and employ LeDoux's (2002) concept of self as "the totality of what an organism is physically, biologically, psychologically, socially and culturally" (31 in Quinn 2006:372). This formulation arises from the understanding that the synaptic activity of "multiple neural systems" works simultaneously "in the process of assembling and maintaining" what we experience as "self" (LeDoux 2002:307). The framework it provides should enable us to avoid the homunculus trap with its associated analytic missteps and develop instead accounts of culture and experience that are "cognitively and neurally realistic" (Lakoff and Johnson 1999:79). As self is all "the totality of what an organism is," to write about identity is merely to demarcate a facet of self-experience for discussion, not to distinguish a separate entity.

Consonant with LeDoux's view of self, my model of the person (and hence my understanding of identity) is, not surprisingly, a cognitive one (Linger 2005) suitable to my use of schema theory. From this perspective, identity may be seen as one or more domains of knowledge about the self formed via associative learning, the putative source of all self-knowledge. Depending upon the circumstances of learning, which may arise from internal as well as external factors, the neural substrate of self-experience may manifest as one identity, or a collection of identities that in turn may be more or less coherent. As there is an element of permanence to such learning, along with constant change, we can expect both to be characteristic of self-understanding. We experience continuity of the self and at the same time, because schema do not prevent us from learning new things, including new things about ourselves, we can also perceive ourselves as in some way transformed.

Given my assumption that intercultural interactions have been a major source of perturbation for Aboriginal people, an assumption that is supported (if not entirely substantiated) by discussions in chapters two and three, it was important for me to look for components of identity that may have arisen from such interactions; contemporary versions of the kind that may have led to Aboriginal rejections of the "wild blackfella" identity of earlier times. It is now widely accepted that ethnic or "race" identities arise from the interaction of groups in possession of distinct cultural histories (for the Australian case see, e.g., Berndt 1977; Hinkson and Smith 2005; Langton 1993; Tonkinson 1990). It is also now widely accepted that invidious comparisons in these identities arise from and accompany whatever social and material inequalities emerge from these encounters (e.g., Cowlishaw 1988; 2004). I think that interactions such as these provide the experiential basis of the facet of identity that may be labeled "Aboriginal person," "blackfella," or *wuruj* [human or person in Wubuy (Heath 1982:295,298)] at Numbulwar. I also think that Aboriginal discourse on whitefellas and on blackfella/whitefella relations may reveal something of what this identity component might be like.

Stories

In line with these assumptions, I asked people at Numbulwar to tell me stories about Aboriginal people and *munangas*, that is, whitefellas. Here I was employing the tactic of giving people a task that likely requires the use of a posited schema (Quinn 2005b:8). In this instance the task consists of requests for stories; the posited schema is that of self-understanding as an Aboriginal person, that is, an "Aboriginal identity."[3] Twelve people, eleven women ranging in age from eighteen to sixty-seven, and one man, a father of two in his late twenties, responded to the first request. Thirteen people, twelve women and the same man, responded to the second. Here is how I framed this task set: (1) Tell me a little story about an Aboriginal person. It can be true or gammon [fantasy/make believe]. (2) Tell me a little story about a *munanga*. It can be true or gammon. What follows is how Majiwi, a woman in her fifties whom readers first encountered in chapter two and heard more from in chapter four, responded. First, she chose to tell a story about Aboriginal people:

> Like there is a group, like my age, like Dahlia and Maya. Like we were learned by one old lady...Dahlia, my sister. She's a real lady that talks and takes the part for the young girl and young boy too.

And [women's names] at the school. It's good what I hear from them, on the loudspeaker. Those two I hear, especially for Dahlia and Suzi, my sister-in-law, and [three more women listed], all teaching at the school. And I hear Dahlia talking to the whole community on the loudspeaker and on the school loudspeaker about children going to school, or maybe they had a Darwin Show; they can't be at the school because they have to take part in it. And maybe they have a holiday. Maria is one of them at the clinic talking to them, like young girls for women's business and at the school, Maria again. Them other ladies, they are teacher for all the children. They are teaching and working on the translation staff. (Majiwi 2003)

Majiwi speaks here of a group of women, more or less her age. Together they were taught, probably at school, by one respected older woman. It is not clear, but I think she is referring to an Aboriginal teaching assistant rather than a whitefella school teacher. Most of these women, at the time of the telling, work at the school as teaching assistants and linguists in the language revival program. Her sister Dahlia, in particular, may, on occasion, use the school's loudspeaker to entreat children to come to school or to make general announcements, such as informing the community that school children will be away, taking part in the Darwin Show, a yearly fair held in Darwin some five hundred kilometers away. Another woman from this group works from the health clinic, providing sex education for adolescent girls. When Majiwi hears the women speaking, she thinks that what they say is "good".

In her second story, Majiwi (2003) chooses to speak about *munanga* who come to Numbulwar:

I can only tell you what I know bout meeting people when they coming in from the city. They need to settle in to Numbulwar. Like they are looking for a job and they would like to come to Numbulwar...Sometime *munanga* see Numbulwar a bad place or good place...Some *munanga* they are good, have really good friendships with people here. And some *munanga* don't listen when we explain things, don't take notice and they get into trouble. They don't listen. If they can take notice, listen to someone who can tell them what word they should not say and tell them not to get wild, then It's OK. I've told many nurses like this, I tell new nurses—she goes to Gove to get orientation, and how she can fit in, nursing, driving, helping people. Maybe she's been in a community before and can move out from there. Maybe they can't take any notice of what we tell them. They get surprised by young people, really young boy [adolescent], breaking into the hospital, bashing car for clinic and stealing car for clinic. And they get scared and ask to be taken away. That's what I've seen in my time when young boy is bashing and taking away hospital vehicle. They break into the clinic and nurse and doctor have to get out for a whole day. And some *munanga*, like in the office, have not been happy there, because they do not take any notice of what people say and just take his path and get in trouble and go away. We had a couple of those staff.

In this story Majiwi has decided to focus on whitefellas who come to Numbulwar. These visitors may have a good or bad opinion of the community. Those who don't like Numbulwar are those who don't pay attention to Aboriginal people when they explain local custom. Interpersonal conflict is the consequence. The actions of these whitefellas may precipitate violent acts that frighten them, even though they are directed against the physical property of the whitefella institution not the staff. These whitefellas leave. In contrast, "good" whitefellas are those who either have previous experience of Aboriginal communities or who are willing to listen to explanations of how things work. These are the whitefellas who "have really good friendship" with Aboriginal people.

There are both parallels in and contrasts between Majiwi's two stories that I find worth exploring. To begin, both are realist accounts of daily life. The first story revolves around Aboriginal women teaching, talking, helping others, and learning. These are activities that take place on a daily basis in this community as they might in any other. They are presented, however, in the manner in which they take place at Numbulwar, for example, over the loudspeaker and at the school. The second story focuses on interactions and events that Majiwi presents herself as being a part of: the reception, orientation, and work trajectory of *munanga* staff. In terms of their realistic aspect, Majiwi's stories are representative of all the other stories collected at Numbulwar from this task set. All of these, both about Aboriginal people and *munanga*s, may be described as realist accounts. Several were explicitly described as "true" by their authors, and the others painted pictures of Aboriginal or *munanga* life that I easily recognized as paralleling if not actually arising from local experiences.

Related to their realist character, both of Majiwi's stories contain what I regard as local content, that is, the stories are uniquely grounded in experiences of Numbulwar, its inhabitants, physical landmarks, and institutions such as the clinic, office, and school. They are also grounded in routine happenings such as announcements on the school loudspeaker and the theft of vehicles. Both stories also contain reference to norms and values of Aboriginal society in this community. For example, in the Aboriginal story, Majiwi is employing at least three culturally specific ideas and alluding to associated values when she says, "Dahlia, my sister. She's a real lady that talks and takes the part for the young girl and young boy too." First she identifies her kin relationship to Dahlia. Talking and taking part (or partner) for someone are actions associated with fighting and nurturing, both of which are expected of kin, especially kin who are in some way seen as responsible for younger people (Burbank 1994), while "young boys" and "young girls" are Kriol terms for adolescents (Burbank 1988). When Majiwi mentions in the *munanga* story "what word they should not say," she could be referring to the requirements of *mirriri*. An example of correct behavior would be remaining silent about a woman's sexual or reproductive functions within the hearing of any man regarded as her brother, something a new nurse unacquainted with Aboriginal etiquette might easily fail to do. Again Majiwi's stories are representative of the total body of stories. All the stories told about Aboriginal people and *munanga*s are constructed out of local content.

Majiwi's two stories also exemplify the contrasts I find between stories told about Aboriginal people and those told about *munangas*. *Munanga*s are relatively rare in stories about Aboriginal people. When they are present, as is the case in four of the twelve stories, they are only mentioned in passing or are given a passive role. The one story about an Aboriginal person in which a *munanga*, the shop manager, plays an active role is as follows:

> I'll tell you about a young boy, he bought this machine in the shop. He saw in the shop a CD and VCR player in one. He wanted to buy it and gave the shop manager $300 and it cost $500 and he told the shop manager he would come back on Friday to pay another $200. But that was on Friday and when he went back on Saturday, the machine was gone. Somebody else bought it. He got his money back and he bought food with the money. And the shop manager said he would order more to come in the barge. (Peg 2003)

In contrast, Aboriginal people are present in all but one of the stories told about *munanga*s. In all of these cases at least one Aboriginal person is presented in an active role. Take, for example, the following fragment. Though the first Aboriginal person to be mentioned, a deceased wife, is clearly a passive actor, others, including the speaker, are then presented in the active role of people asking questions:

> George, he's a white man...He's married to a Traditional Owner here [someone with a father/child link to the country upon which Numbulwar is located], That's George's wife and we been ask him after she died, "What your life gonna be? You going back to your family?" (Vikki 2003)

Majiwi and this speaker are not alone in including themselves in stories about *munanga*s. A total of five storytellers put themselves in these stories, all presenting themselves in a positive if not heroic light:

> Some *munanga* good, some bad, some polite. [Bad *munanga*] they don't talk, get real stressed out quick. And if Aboriginal people, they do anything wrong, break and enter school teacher houses, they call to the police. I've been helping *munanga*, helping them all my life. *Munanga* went to their home and found everything, DVD, tape, money gone. Me and my husband we are here for them. We drive around every day checking each teacher house when they go away. (Emma 2005)

At the end of one of the school holidays in 2005, several school teachers returning to Numbulwar discovered that their houses had been broken into during their absence and items such as tape recorders, DVD players, and money taken. The police had been called in to discover the culprits and recover the items if possible. In her story, Emma refers to this set of events, casting herself, and her husband, as protectors of teachers' property.

Western readers unacquainted with Numbulwar might not recognize a positive self-presentation in the following:

> *Munanga*, Eddie, school teacher. He used to be riding around, joking might be. Him run run...run down and all around the school and I was going to my aunty's place and I saw this man and I ask him question, "What for you doing this?" And he told me, "I do exercise because I'm going to Athens, Olympics." He is going to Athens for the sport. He wanted to win that trophy. You can see him on Saturday. He's a good runner he told me. He wanted to go to that Olympics. That's true story. And I told him, "What that sport?" And he answer, "One hundred meter." That's all he told me. (Merry 2004)

However, people familiar with the sense of standing implied in at least some Aboriginal communities by the ability to ask a question of someone, and receive an answer (see von Strumer 1981), even a humorous one, might interpret this as I do, that is, as a presentation of self highlighting one's equal, if not higher, position vis-à-vis a whitefella school teacher.

Given a minimal presence of *munangas* in Aboriginal stories, in contrast to the presence of Aboriginal people in *munanga* stories, it is not surprising that I find discussions of blackfella/whitefella relationships and interaction largely in the latter. I think that the tone of these relationships and interactions is highly relevant for understanding Aboriginal identity. Three of the storytellers presented only positive accounts. An example of a positive *munanga* story comes from the male storyteller:

> We had a whitefella here, came here and sit with us and we had a little talk; he made friends with us. We always take him out and he always has fun with us. Sometime he feels so lonely he comes with us and sits with us and we have a yarn. Like what's gonna be happening here. And we went with that whitefella to place called [place name] and he came there with us. We took him for two weeks and he told us, "I like this place, beautiful place. I can stay here all of my life." Sometimes he tell us white people they don't talk together because he likes Aboriginal people, he don't like white people. And we had a lot of fun at the plain with that whitefella and we came back home on Monday. (Gerard 2003)

A visiting whitefella became friends with Gerard and his family. He visits them, they have fun together, and recently they took him to Gerard's mother's country, which the whitefella admired. The whitefella tells Gerard that some whitefellas don't talk to him; he prefers to socialize with Aboriginal people and "don't like" whites. This comment, assuming it reflects something the whitefella actually said, could be the whitefella's way of distinguishing himself from other whitefellas. If such is the case it's hard to know if the strategy arose from observations of Aboriginal dislike of "white people" or from a possibly mistaken belief that this might be the case. Of course, this man may have genuinely disliked the other whitefellas in residence at Numbulwar. Speculation aside, of greatest relevance for the discussion to follow in this and subsequent chapters is the fact that dislike of white people is included in a story that highlights an intercultural friendship.

Three other speakers presented negative stories, an example of which follows:

> Some *munanga* do not like talking and do not like Aboriginal people. Some *munanga* they like some baskets and maybe necklace and some spears and, you know, that turtle shell. [They do not like Aboriginal people] because they are too silly and they go to them for money and want to sell this one and they tell Aboriginal people to go back home now. That school teacher he growls at kids, tell them to go to school and not to come to school, to go home. He is angry one. They don't like him now. They want education, to learn more. That teacher talks to kids rough way and makes you upset and they go tell parents to go to the school and talk to the principal. They want education, they want to learn more. And then they grow up they work to school, office, respite [center caring for the aged and disabled], homeland [center servicing several small settlements associated with Numbulwar]. (Sherry 2003)

According to Sherry, some whitefellas "do not like" Aboriginal people and "do not like talking" with them. They might, however, like the things they peddle from door to door. Here Sherry appears to see some justification in *munanga* dislike of Aboriginal people "because they are too silly," which implies that peddling is a form of misbehavior; it may not simply be experienced as an annoying intrusion but as a form of harassment. This entrepreneurial activity was usually understood by both blackfellas and whitefellas as driven by a need for ganja. In contrast, the school teacher is simply an angry, aggressive person who upsets people because he speaks harshly to their children. When they misbehave in class he sends them home. He reprimands them "rough way" when they don't come to school and tells their parents to see the school principal about their children's behavior. He doesn't recognize that Aboriginal people value learning and education and the employment that might follow.

Like Majiwi, three other storytellers included both positive and negative relationships and interactions in their stories; for example, a young woman storyteller said:

> Some *munanga* they don't like Aboriginal people. Some *munanga* like Aboriginal people. Teach them more English, Batchelor [College] study. They can teach their children when they come back from Batchelor. They will be with their parents. And if they grow up they'll be in high school in Darwin in Australia. And they come back and they teach when they have kids. (Raelene 2003)

Like Sherry, Raelene says that some whitefellas don't like Aboriginal people. She makes it clear, however, that the category "whitefella" is one that does not prevent at least some Aboriginal people from differentiating among them. Whitefellas are not seen as a homogeneous mass. Some don't like Aboriginal people, but others do. Those who do like them, teach them. Here Raelene is talking about the English language teaching that takes place at the Batchelor Institute of Indigenous Tertiary Education, located about one hundred kilometers south of Darwin and usually referred to by its old name, Batchelor College. This teaching enables Aboriginal people to do further study in Darwin high schools and, upon their return to Numbulwar, to teach their own children.

Strikingly, three storytellers told *munanga* stories that did not include relationships or interactions between Aboriginal people and *munanga*. One of these stories had no Aboriginal characters in it. In the two others, while both Aboriginal people and *munanga*s are present, they do not interact, nor are they cast in any relationship. Here is one of these stories:

> *Munanga*, him live in a house and it's different to Aboriginal people, Indigenous people. They live the way they have been taught. It's their way, what their family been teaching them to live, and they cook the way they cook and they sleep the way they sleep in the bunk. They do their shopping and put it in the fridge and keep it there and they use money really good way, not like Aboriginal people use money. *Munanga* is different, they live, they cook, they look after themselves and they buy everything they need, maybe, probably before the weekend. They don't waste money like Aboriginal people waste money. Right? (Lily 2003)

Lily takes a noticeably anthropological perspective on *munanga*s in this text. They live in a way that may be distinguished from an Aboriginal way because they have been taught to live that way. She does not, however, take a relativistic stance when she compares their respective ways of handling money, unless "waste" does not have the same meaning for her that it does for me. As we will see later in this chapter, Lily and I appear to share similar views on waste.

All the stories include statements about interactions that are seen as either appropriate or pleasurable or as inappropriate or wrong and are valued or devalued accordingly. The following Aboriginal story illustrates the inclusion of both valued and devalued interactions:

> I'll tell you story about us mob, we been go fishing, me and [two women]. We went to collect mussels, *warlgu* [mussels], at the jungle there. We was collecting maybe ten, twenty *warlgu* and cooking them

on the fire. At 3:00 we came back and we saw this buffalo standing by the tree. And after we saw the buffalo we saw a woman, collecting pandanus, [a third woman named]. I don't know how that buffalo didn't chase her. And we told her, "Buffalo there," and to go back with us, but she didn't listen. She wanted to collect pandanus for making baskets. And after she was angry with us, growling at us. And we left her there and we came back here, we went back home now. That true story one. (Merry 2004)

Merry and her companions went up the coast for a day of fishing and gathering at a place some distance from town. On their return trip they saw a feral water buffalo, an animal justly feared by Aboriginal people, especially when they are in the bush on foot. When they saw another woman who appears to have been alone, a highly unusual circumstance for a woman on a gathering expedition, they informed her of its presence and offered to accompany her back to Numbulwar. Rather than accept their offer she spoke angrily to the group of women, who then left her and continued on their way. The woman gathering pandanus suffers from a chronic mental illness, which most likely accounts for her solitary gathering. It also probably accounts for her hostile response, although Merry attributes a desire to make baskets as her motive for staying in the bush alone and for "growling" at the other women. Neither gathering alone nor responding to offers of help with anger is typical behavior.

Statements about women fishing, gathering, and cooking together, providing helpful information and the offer of protection to another person are clearly about positive forms of interaction. In contrast, the description of a woman not listening to others, especially when they are being helpful, and speaking harshly to them, is clearly about negative forms of interaction. Overall, the tone of the interactions in the *munanga* stories is notably less positive than that of the Aboriginal stories. The Aboriginal stories include statements about more than thirty-eight positive interactions and only fifteen negative ones. In contrast, the *munanga* stories have a near balance of positive and negative interactions between Aboriginal people and *munanga*, twenty and twenty-four, respectively.

As with accounts of interactions, words or phrases describing emotions or feelings may be described as positive or negative, given my acquaintance with their meanings to the people employing them. Words such as "wild," "scared," "angry," and "upset" describe states that people of Numbulwar find unpleasant and devalue as can be seen in several of the stories , as well as from the analysis of words associated with stress in chapter four. Similarly, words such as "like" and phrases such as "have fun" indicate valued feelings, as the story by Gerard presented earlier in this section illustrates. The *munanga* stories include negative emotions and feelings more than twice as often as they include positive ones, nineteen to eight. The Aboriginal stories are more balanced, including as they do eight negative descriptors and twelve positive ones.[4]

Majiwi's two stories exemplify this contrast of tone. Her stories also exemplify many of the others insofar as they include explicit evaluations of people and their actions. This is particularly the case in her *munanga* story. Some of the evaluations in the stories come directly from the storyteller as when Majiwi says, "Some *munanga* they are good, have really good friendships with people here." In other cases, a story's actor is made to do the evaluating as when Merry has Eddie the school teacher describe himself as "a good runner." Nine of the *munanga* stories included such explicit evaluations of *munangas*: six of the storytellers evaluated *munangas* directly, three indirectly.

Aboriginal people, their community or their culture, are also evaluated in the *munanga* stories as when Majiwi says, "Sometime *munanga* see Numbulwar a bad place, or good place." Seven of the stories include such evaluations. Again, these may be those of the storyteller as when one describes people stealing from *munanga* as "silly," as mentioned, a word used to label someone engaged in misbehavior. Three stories include direct evaluations of Aboriginal people. More often, in five cases, Aboriginal people or their culture are evaluated by *munangas*: "He always tells my husband, 'I'm white, but I've got no life but for Aboriginal'" (Vikki 2003). Only two *munanga* stories do not contain any explicitly evaluative content. One of these is the only *munanga* story that does not have an Aboriginal actor in it. The other story with no explicit evaluative content comes from another woman in her late fifties, Ngalba (2003):

> A whitefella saw a young boy walking carrying tape [gesture of holding tape recorder on shoulder]. And he took his tape after he got off work and now he was carrying that tape [again gesture of tape recorder on shoulder]. He was walking with that tape on his shoulder to the beach, like young boy. That man, he was a pilot, putting loud music, walking down the beach. We saw him and said, "That one, he's acting like those young fellas."

After seeing an adolescent boy carrying a tape recorder on his shoulder, a whitefella pilot, stationed at Numbulwar, did the same, playing it at a high volume while he walked to the beach. Ngalba and her companions saw him and remarked that he was acting like the adolescent boys. While there is no explicit evaluative content in Ngalba's story, it doesn't seem much of a stretch to see an implicit evaluation in it. On the one hand, Aboriginal practice, that of young boys carrying their tape recorders on their shoulders, is worthy of emulation. On the other, such behavior on the part of young boys is greeted, at best, with ambivalence by people the age of Ngalba. When she has people say, "That one, he's acting like those young fellas," she renders the pilot's act as an imitative one and implicitly judges his behavior as immature.

In the Aboriginal stories, evaluation, though present, is much less apparent. In only five cases do I feel confident making this identification. The most clear cut example of an evaluative component in a story about Aboriginal people is as follows: "Those young people, they breaking things all right, breaking windows, stealing things, only boys. Not the girls, girls good, not doing these things. Only some of the girls are stealing" (Wilwila 2003). In Wilwila's story adolescent boys are breaking windows and stealing. Adolescent girls, however are "good," they are "not doing these things," except for "some" who "are stealing." Even here, however, it is not the boys' actions that are labeled "bad." Instead, it is girls who are "good" because they are not breaking windows and stealing.

The other stories similarly detail actions that I know are generally regarded as good and bad. For example, Aboriginal stories include accounts of people making mistakes, talking too much, running around, and making loud noises at night when people are trying to sleep, frightening people, and performing "black magic." All of these are actions that adults, such as the storytellers, would likely say are "bad" if asked directly. Yet none are labeled bad, nor are the people who perform them. Valued actions are more common in these stories—actions such as hunting and sharing, helping, knowing how to ride a horse, reciprocating, telling stories, laughing, and having fun. But none of these actions or their originators is labeled as good. In none of the stories about Aboriginal people is a *munanga* evaluated.

Aboriginal Identity

It is this latter contrast between Aboriginal and *munanga* stories that I think especially telling for that component of self-understanding we call Aboriginal identity. Logically, Aboriginal identity arises in interaction with non-Aboriginal people and as these stories suggest, these have been interactions infused with an evaluative component. Identification of this component of Aboriginal identity begins to explain a pattern of response that I received to another question about Aboriginal identity. I asked this of sixteen people, fourteen women and two men, including most of those I asked to tell me stories about Aboriginal and *munanga* people. Here is the question: "How do you feel yourself about being an Aboriginal person in Australia these days?"

Twelve of the respondents used words such as "proud" and "good," indicating that understanding oneself as an Aboriginal person frequently involves a self-evaluation, as the following two responses illustrate.

> I like being an Aboriginal person. I'm Aboriginal girl because I'm black, got my mother, father, grandmother, grandfather, they all black, Aboriginal people. So I can learn my culture, what it means to me. Because it means everything to me, Aboriginal way. Especially the ceremony. I want to be that way, Aboriginal girl, person. (Merry 2004)

> Well, I'm really happy about it, to be an Indigenous person, because I live in my country and I live with [pause]. I'm understanding every-thing in my culture, the way my ancestors used to live and learning more about things way way back. When I was a little girl, I was learning about culture and place, places and how we been related and how we been—the stories and country and the way we been living at bush. Our ancestors, old people been teaching us the way we been living long time ago and what we've been doing, hunting and every year and every month we've been staying at bush. Now these days it's different, it's different now because we don't go bush anymore, we stay all the time in town, but we go out fishing, hunting still, we have ceremony, dancing, we have culture day for the children at the school and they teach them at the school and we have language, they teach them at the school, and when they come down to the Village, we speak to them in Nunggubuyu and some can understand, some can't. They still know how they are related. Some understand, some don't. Things are changing. It's really, you know, some of our old people still alive. (Lily 2003)

Even with my follow-up question, "Any bad things about being an Aboriginal person?," there were only seven respondents who offered, usually brief, comments on negative aspects of Aboriginality. Here is

Ngalba's (2003) response:

> *Ngalba*: We feel good that we are, what do you callit, Indigenous person, like we are proud of ourself.
> *VKB*: When you are thinking about yourself as an Aboriginal person, are there times you feel bad?
> *Ngalba*: Like sometimes, when *munanga* say bad things about Aboriginal people, we feel bad.

In 2004, when I returned to Numbulwar I spoke with Ngalba again and asked her to tell me a story about "a bad *munanga*."[5] This is the story Ngalba (2004) then told and the conversation we had about it:

> *Ngalba*: *Munanga*, she do it her own way. She doesn't listen to what Aboriginal people want. Sometime she's good, but sometime she doesn't want what they, Aboriginal people, want. She wants to do it her own way of doing. She's not really bad, she gets along alright, but sometime she doesn't take notice of them when they say something to her, she take notice of others. She doesn't, they work with her, Aboriginal people, but she doesn't listen, she does her own way and if you want her to do something she runs it her own way. If you tell her something to do, she won't do it. She do it her way. More better she reckon than Aboriginal way. That's what all the *munanga* reckon. Aboriginal got no better idea. *Munanga* think ahead, maybe Aboriginal crazy one. *Munanga* make mistake too.
> *VKB*: When you think about her, how do you feel?
> *Ngalba*: I feel bad.

In Ngalba's two responses we can see a connection between how one feels about oneself as an Aboriginal person and how *munanga*s can make one feel, feelings that may be dissonant. When Ngalba thinks about herself as an "Indigenous person" she feels proud. However, when she hears *munanga*s saying "bad things" about Aboriginal people she feels bad. When a whitefella ignores her advice she not only feels bad about herself, she also transforms a single *munanga*'s attitude toward her into a general *munanga* attitude toward Aboriginal people: the *munanga* who thinks Aboriginal "got no better idea" become "all the *munanga*" who think this.[6] Both of Ngalba's responses also continue the evaluative emphasis in the *munanga* stories.

While much of the evaluation of the *munanga* stories involves the speaker evaluating a *munanga*, I propose that this process once introduced works both ways; indeed the evaluation of *munanga*s as good and bad may be a response to being evaluated by *munanga*s as good or bad Aboriginal people. For example, here is another question that I asked of eleven people to activate an Aboriginal identity schema and Lily's (2004) reply:

> *VKB*: What do you think *munanga* think about Aboriginal people these days?
> *Lily*: Some *munanga* say Aboriginal people, you know, they are good. Some *munanga* say they are bad. When they think about people in Gove, Katherine, Darwin, everywhere else, not here. They don't like to see them, drinkers in Darwin, they don't like to see them; they like to send them back to their community. When white [people] see Aboriginal people in Darwin, they are wondering what makes them stay in Darwin, drink in Darwin. They don't like to go back to their country, go to the bush... [Munanga think], well some people, maybe these people are good and they are learning what we are teaching, right way. But some people not doing the right way, drinking too much, smoking too much [ganja]. And they see a lot of drunken people, tell them to go away, not to come where they live. Some people don't like them; some *munanga* don't like Aboriginal people because they drinking and fighting, they don't want them to stay around town, especially in Darwin. They want them to come back to their own land and family... When we go to Darwin, they ask us for one dollar, two dollar. When we don't have money we don't give them. When we have money we give them one dollar, two dollar. Not only *munanga* don't like them, Aborigine don't like them because they wasting money when they get paid. White and black don't like people that drink.

There are, according to Lily, two different opinions of Aboriginal people that various *munanga* hold. There are bad and good Aboriginal people. There is something familiar about this dichotomy; it reminds me of the contrast that Ngalakan speakers have drawn between "wild blackfellas" and "station blacks," mentioned in chapter three. This contrast, according to Morphy and Morphy (1984), likely originated in the stereotypes of Aboriginal people that white settlers both held and broadcast. Its historical and geographic pervasiveness in the region is suggested by its use in a report on the Roper River Mission at the turn of the last century:

> Beside the Mission children, there are wild blacks who often camp nearby. Any Aboriginal can get food, tobacco, and clothing, provided he or she works for it, and much of the labour on the station is done

by these wild blacks, such as digging the irrigation channels and herd-
ing the goats. The wild blacks come and go, and the Mission does not
attempt to instruct or educate them. They describe themselves to outsiders as Mission Blacks but are not regarded by the Missionaries as
such (Masson 1913 in Morphy and Morphy 1984:471).

"Wild blacks" then were nomads, not to be educated or instructed.
Wild blacks today, that is, bad Aboriginal people according to Lily's
scheme, are those who stay in town to drink, smoke ganja, and
waste money. In contrast, good Aboriginal people are those who
learn the "right way" from *munanga*s, just as station blacks were
those whose loyalty and labor once made whitefellas' Roper Valley
stations (ranches) viable concerns.

When Lily comments of drinkers in her story that "Not only
munanga don't like them, Aborigine don't like them because they
wasting money when they get paid. White and black don't like people that drink," I begin to wonder about the extent to which her own
opinions about some Aboriginal people at least are being presented
as *munanga*s' views. I also begin to ask if this may not represent a
greater degree of identification with *munanga*s than is first apparent in this story, and if such identification is the case, how it might
reverberate in her self-understanding.

Like Lily, other respondents to this question saw bad and good
Aboriginal people through *munanga* eyes; and most of the discussion of the other ten respondents was, like Lily's, reserved for detail-
ing a negative view of Aboriginal people:

> What do *munanga* think about us? Some *munanga* think we bring
> problems in cities, like people live in cities, they walk around drunken,
> sleep in the grass by the side of the road. They think we are hopeless;
> we not got enough to look after ourself. (Peg 2003)

> Like *munanga* thinking some Aboriginal people don't learn maybe,
> learn more education, experience for work. Because Aborigine go
> behind *munanga*. Instead of this land is for Aborigines. But white
> people go first. And Aboriginal people listen to *munanga*, what they
> gonna do, like for work. And cleaning. And last year they had that, like
> each house gonna have lawn and fences and work for CDP and young
> boy should clean up boundaries and owner should clean up inside the
> boundaries and *munanga* put the fence. Also for dog. That vet maybe
> coming over here, only one dog, people are going to be allowed to
> have, because some dogs got scabies and sores. (Sunny 2003)

> Whitefella think when they look at Aboriginal people, they think he
> doesn't understand anything. Maybe he does not speak English well,

understand *munanga* way. Maybe *munanga* might think, "Dumb one. He doesn't know anything." Like here if you gotta job and you can't handle that job, can't cope with everything you have to do, "Oh he doesn't know, him dumb. He doesn't know." (Ngalba 2003)

Peg, Sunny, and Ngalba, a relatively young woman in her early thirties, a middle-aged woman, and an old woman, respectively, all from different clans and different households, share some of their ideas about what whitefellas think of blackfellas. In particular, all three women say that *munangas* think they are unintelligent and incapable of taking responsibility for their own lives, that "we not got enough to look after ourself," that "Aboriginal people don't learn" and need to "listen to munanga, what they gonna do." They are people that "doesn't know," people that are "dumb."

With only one exception, all of the responses to this question presented negative views of Aboriginal people or rejection of Aboriginal people in *munanga* thought.[7] I suggest that just as the Aboriginal and *munanga* stories are realist accounts of life at Numbulwar, so these responses are based on experiences their speakers have had or know about.

A catalog of the harmful consequences of domination includes the internalization of derogatory treatment, the potential becoming of one as inferior as one is thought to be (e.g., Fanon 1967; Memmi 1957; Sennett and Cobb 1972). Assuming that the comments presented earlier are representative of those that could be made by any other Aboriginal person at Numbulwar, Aboriginal identity may well include, though not be limited to, perceptions of self as hopeless, unable to care for oneself, subordinate to *munangas* in matters as intimate as housekeeping, unable to speak English fluently, ignorant and dumb. Looking at remarks found in the other responses, the Aboriginal component of self for many people at Numbulwar may also include feelings that whitefellas don't "like" or want to be physically close to people of "we color."

At this point readers might question the seeming equation of these texts with the speakers' self-understanding. Is it not possible to speak about negative characteristics of Aboriginal people without believing that the self also possesses them? I argue here that insofar as the authors of these texts identify themselves as Aboriginal people, these characteristics are a part of their self-understanding, but in varying ways and to varying degrees. Take, for example, Lily's discussion of bad Aboriginal people as "drinkers." Knowing she is not a drinker, we may suppose that her self-understanding includes this fact. We might thus represent "bad Aboriginal drinker" as the "not me" part of her self schema (see Gregg 1998; Kakar 1996). But what of Ngalba's characterization of Aboriginal people as dumb? Although I have argued that negative feelings may be minimized to some extent by local child rearing practice, it is difficult to imagine anyone who has not experienced subordination, insult, and unwelcomed control by others, if only because all humans necessarily go through varying periods of physical and emotional dependency. All experiences of this order might be internalized in terms of a self that is dumb, ignorant, and helpless. The extent to which these experiences permeate self-understanding, however, undoubtedly differs.

Why do some things that we learn about ourselves become more central than other things? Learning that occurs early in our development, particularly when it is accompanied by a moderate degree of emotional arousal, is thought to be both enduring and motivational (Strauss and Quinn 1997). It follows that early and emotional lessons about ourselves are enduring and motivational in our sense of who we are and want to be (D'Andrade 1992; Quinn 2005c; Strauss and Quinn 1997). Many Aboriginal people at Numbulwar likely begin to learn about themselves as Aboriginal people quite early on. For example, one of my more disconcerting experiences at Numbulwar, repeated more often than I would like, and one I no doubt share with other *munangas* who have lived there, is that of being used to frighten or discipline children. As a stranger, and perhaps a particularly strange one given my light skin color, small children have sometimes begun to cry or whimper upon my approach. Typically, the child's mother or caretaker would envelop the child in her arms while saying something along the lines of, "*Bamudarba* [be quiet], *munanga* there." In these instances children have been directed to control themselves, protected by a familiar Aboriginal person and warned of a frightening stranger, labeled "*munanga.*" Such lessons likely continue as the child is taken to the clinic, where the *munanga* may be the person who both frightens and hurts the child, and at school where for the first time the child may experience their most sustained separation from familiar caretakers. It seems reasonable to assume that the Aboriginal person component of identity, as "not *munanga,*" is a part of people's core self-understanding.

Did a *munanga* ever call Ngalba dumb? Did she hear about a *munanga* calling another Aboriginal person dumb? Or did Ngalba, having been told that she couldn't handle "a job," which is a *munanga* thing, or thinking that she couldn't handle a job, label herself as dumb. Whatever the origin, she has made an association between

Aboriginal people and being dumb. However, we do not know if this characterization of Aboriginal people characterizes Ngalba to herself. What kind of experience could make her do so? As a child she might or might not have felt dumb as a Wubuy speaker with an English speaking teacher. She might simply have experienced herself as a person who did not speak the teacher's language. What if not speaking English as a young child in school led to the frustration of a desire, say, for a teacher's approval or a reward? The emotional concomitant of the experience of being dumb, especially if repeated over time, might well give "dumb" a pride of place in Ngalba's understanding of herself as an Aboriginal person.

Frustration of Desires

In assuming that people's identity contents may ameliorate or exacerbate the extent to which stress has harmful effects on bodies and minds, I join a number of other scholars who have conceptualized links between the ways we feel about ourselves and our health and well-being. Three efforts in particular closely resemble the way I have been thinking about identity and ill health.

The first of these, closely linked with the social determinants of health framework, is represented by a study undertaken by Demakakos and his team (2008) who have looked at the effects that a "subjective social status" may have had on the health of a sample consisting of thousands of older people, age fifty-two and above, in the English population. An assumption of their study is that "subjective social status" (SSS), the way people see their own position relative to that of others in a social hierarchy, is associated in some manner with what they call "objective indicators of SES," that is, "wealth, occupational class and education" (332). Their findings indicate that our relative sense of socioeconomic status can indeed be identified as a risk to our health. In particular, their interpretation suggests that it is these perceptions that "mediate" the effects of education and occupational class. That is to say, education and occupational class affect our health because the more likely we are to be well educated and not only gainfully but also prestigiously employed, the more likely we are to see ourselves occupying a relatively high position in the socioeconomic hierarchy. And this kind of self-perception is good for us. Wealth, however, did not act in this way to the same extent. Though overlapping with SSS, it had some independent effect on health. Here, however, gender differences are apparent; wealth having more of an independent effect on the health of men than that of women. Demakakos and his colleagues specu-late that:

> These differences might reflect gender differences in the mean-ing of achievement in life and need to be considered in the light of the different ways that men and women understand the world and evaluate their life-time successfulness. For the women of our cohort life-time achievement might be less economic in nature than for the men. (335)

At least to an anthropological eye, Demakakos et al. (2008) intro-duce the possibility of different cultural values mediating the effects of "objective" factors in their conjecture about gender-specific understandings and evaluations of life accomplishments, for we can take gender to be a point of social disjunction across which facets of cultural understanding may not be shared (e.g., Gilligan 1982). Thus we can see how "objective" factors may cease to be objec-tive, at least across cultural boundaries, in a most material way, the capacity to affect human physiology.

The second effort that resembles the way I have been thinking about identity and ill health is Agar and Reisinger's (2001) attempt to understand heroin epidemics. The idea of "open marginality" describes a historical moment where "change had produced an unexpected and dramatic difference between expectations and real-ity for some part of the population," usually one that is circum-scribed by a marginalized, minority identity (Agar 2003:25). The difference between expectations and reality is due to changes either in expectations or in reality; expectations may be, unrealistically, raised or life gets worse, in part because of attention that powerful others pay to the minority group. That is to say, when government policy and media spotlights focus on particular identities, the gap may be exacerbated not least because public discourses reconfigure the minority identity, often by delineating and emphasizing negative characteristics associated with it. This exacerbates a tension of par-ticular relevance to my approach: the marginalized identity, while valued by the marginalized group, is devalued even less than previ-ously by the superordinate group.

A third approach bearing similarities to mine is found in an overview of psychosocial stress models used to understand "racial and ethnic health disparities" (Dressler et al. 2005:203) and vari-ous attempts to identify "the specific ethnographic realities" of social inequalities that generate health-damaging stress in African American lives. Dressler et al. find a pattern that may be described as the mismatch of aspirations and the means to achieve them. When we are repeatedly frustrated because our resources provide us with inadequate means for achieving valued goals, there is a greater likelihood we will experience relative deprivation, harmful stress, and consequent ill health. Dressler (1991a) has pursued this direction in health research via the concept of "lifestyle incongruity," the "degree to which an individual's lifestyle exceeds his or her socioeconomic status (occupation combined with education)" (611). In developing this concept, he has drawn on Veblen's (1918) idea that: "To gain and to hold the esteem of men it is not sufficient merely to possess wealth or power. The wealth or power must be put in evidence" (Veblen 1918:36 in Dressler 1990:184). Driving a "nice" car and living in a nice house in a good neighborhood are examples of the kinds of displays of material wealth that may be required to gain the esteem of one's fellows in an American middle-class context. At the time and place of Dressler's studies, few of the promises of the American civil rights movement had been realized; many disadvantaged African Americans had neither the standard of education nor the level of employment that would enable them to acquire the accoutrements of "success." Instead, they had been left "struggling to maintain a conventional middle-class lifestyle in the context of low socioeconomic status" (Dressler 1991a:611), what in a past era might have been called "living beyond their means," a condition long found shameful, at least by an elite segment of American society (e.g., Wharton 1966). The correlations found in Dressler's (1990; 1991b) studies provide support for the idea that "lifestyle incongruity" is "a potent risk factor" for mental and physical ill health. Dressler (1991a) proposes that an individual experiencing more rather than less incongruence "may be hypervigilant in social interaction, attempting to 'convince' others...of his or her true status" (612).

For Dressler, a lower status, or devalued identity, appears as the precursor to frustration. In contrast, I see frustration as both a precursor and an accompaniment of a negative identity component, though I would note that Dressler's views and mine are not mutually exclusive. I suggest that the frustration of desire is an emotional experience that strengthens the associations that many Aboriginal people have made between being an Aboriginal person and characteristics they have been taught to devalue. We can begin to see that some forms of identity, those that both arise from and exacerbate goal frustration, may be, in and of themselves, sources of stress and subsequent ill health. Given their invidious sources, we are directed to look for desires or goals arising from the *munanga* world.

Big Things

The original inhabitants of Numbulwar, several of whom provided some of the texts presented in this chapter and in chapter four, were pushed and pulled into the realm of the *munanga*s, or at least their parents were. They were pushed by the missions and perhaps by fear of violence from whitefella or Aboriginal intruders in their land. They were pulled by their desires to live apart from their enemies and to consume tobacco, if not sugar and flour (Burbank 1980). I asked fifteen people, most of whom also answered the questions designed to tap Aboriginal identity, about aspects of life at Numbulwar that they thought were good or would make the "best life for people at Numbulwar in the years ahead." The answers to these questions, along with my observations of contemporary life in the town, suggest that the push and pull toward *munanga* life continues today. All but two replies included Western items or ideas. The replies of Merry and Sherry, both mothers of school-aged children, provide a nice matched set of illustrations of how Western culture intrudes in what might be described as a desire for a fairly "traditional" lifestyle:

> Enjoying yourself. Going hunting, showing kids how to collect bush tucker and sea food. Learning kids how to play sport. Learning, schooling, education. Going to outstation and show kids whose country this is. That's the good life. (Merry 2004)

> Good things. They like to watch TV. Go fishing, camping out, they want to, like to, get to killing turtle and dugong. Make them happy. And they like to go to the beach. (Sherry 2003)

Even with an emphasis on hunting and fishing, "killing turtle and dugong," the "good life" includes "sport," "schooling," and "TV."

There can be little doubt that people at Numbulwar have long seen an attraction in much of the West's material culture. In Western terms, however, most of the people at Numbulwar are "poor people" living off of various forms of "welfare." Because of the ubiquitous practice of "demand sharing" (Peterson 1993), even the few people with jobs and salaries commensurate with those of middle-class Australians must scramble to save money for desired items and then struggle to maintain them when they are acquired. The ethnographic literature on Aboriginal Australia abounds with examples of conflicts and frustrations associated with the desire for expensive and not so expensive items of Western material culture (e.g., Austin-Broos 2003; Myers 1988; Sharp 1952). The following exchange that I had with the teenager Kinsey (2005), suggests not only the tensions associated with material acquisitions but their association with *munangas*, not Aborigines:

> *VKB*: Did you ever wish to be a *munanga*?
> *Kinsey*: No. Yeh. Sometimes.
> *VKB*: Really?
> *Kinsey*: No. I just want to be like Aboriginal because we got Aboriginal color, like brown color.
> *VKB*: Did you ever dream you were a *munanga*?
> *Kinsey*: No. Not really. If you want to make yourself *munanga*, you want to buy everything, to make yourself famous. Everybody do that here. Make themself famous. Buy big thing like truck, TV, video. That's why they call them *munanga* because they buy big thing. Everything they buy. That's why they call them famous. They reckon themselves pretty and nice.

Kinsey's metaphorical use of the phrases "make yourself *munanga*" and "make themselves famous" to talk about specific consumptions practices signals to me the introduction of a pointed and potent status difference into the relatively egalitarian Aboriginal domain. This kind of status difference clearly originates in a comparison of the material wealth of whitefellas and blackfellas. The possible consequences of such consumption practices, or the desire for such consumption, that Kinsey does not mention are the frustrations that inevitably follows. Because these are associated with identity and inequality, they are likely to be more rather than less emotive. Hence, according to what we understand about schema, they are also likely to lead to devalued characteristics gaining strength in Aboriginal people's sense of self. Thus, Lily does not restrict "wasting money" to bad Aboriginal people: "*Munanga* is different, they live, they cook, they look after themselves and they buy everything they need, maybe, probably before the weekend. They don't waste money like Aboriginal people waste money. Right?" (Lily 2003). Kinsey and Lily, one young woman, one old, appear to be sharing a similar train of thought. People who are able to buy "big thing" may be "pretty and nice," but people who are not may be bad Aboriginal people, always, "wasting money" and of course even people who may buy a video one day are people who may not buy a truck or an iPod the next. Not having big things can make people feel bad about themselves not simply as people who cannot achieve something they desire but as Aboriginal people.

All Stars

Shortly after my return to Numbulwar in 2004 I had the following conversation with a woman in her early twenties:

> VKB: Do you have TV?
> AW: Yes and I just bought All Stars. It was put on Wednesday. On Monday, I have to buy a new TV with a big screen. It [All Stars] has 999 channels.
> VKB: How much does it cost?
> AW: $200. They took it out of my account.
> VKB: Is that one off?
> AW: Yes. (2004:III:2–3)

According to *munanga* residents at Numbulwar, something like $200 was the connection charge. There was also a monthly fee. The amount of this depended upon the chosen program, the least expensive of which was around $50. By 2005 at least three women that I know had lost their All Stars:

> Sherry shows me a piece of cardboard with a [phone] number written on it and [the figure] $646.50. "I gotta ask you to help me with this one. Maybe you can give me $50 or $100." This is what she owes All Stars, that is, what she has to pay before they will turn it back on. They turned it off. She is going to put $100 and $100 and $100, counts $100 six times and $40 and $6 and fifty cents. "That's not hard." She has given All Stars her mobile number and they will call her (when they turn it back on). Says other people have to pay All Stars, maybe $600, $700, $800, $900. (2005:V:66–7)

> I've got DVD. I got TV. I got All Stars, but they turned it off. But I'm going to pay and get it back on. I like watching TV the most, All Stars. They got lots of movie, make you stay home when they put All Stars. I didn't like to walk around or go visit family, cause I like All Stars. All sorts of movie. Best movie, like all sorts of channels. (Misha 2005)

Sherry and Misha seemed to accept their debt with equanimity, perhaps because they had not yet begun to pay it off. Merry's experience, however, was of a different order. On one very hot afternoon in December, a "pay day" when welfare checks were paid into people's accounts, Merry thought she had finally paid off her All Stars debt and would soon have the service reconnected. This might have been especially important to her because one of her school-aged sons liked to watch it; reconnecting All Stars would be an act very much in keeping with expectations about good mothering (Burbank 2006; Burbank and Chisholm 1989). Merry rang All Stars on her mobile only to be told, after a long conversation, that she still owed $700, though according to her reckoning she had paid them $1000. "I'm going to give them argument," she said and started talking about the receipts she had for her payments, and how someone at the Credit Union had been "stealing" her money. To me, her anger, disappointment and distress were palpable; I thought I might even be seeing a dangerous rise in her blood pressure as her face seemed to swell and the sweat dripped from her brow.[8]

Here, I think, is an example of ill health in the making. We can empathize with Merry, imagining first her long call to All Stars, perhaps being transferred from desk to desk, getting an answer she neither anticipated nor believed. Who among us has not been suspended in webs of meaning someone else has spun, especially on telephone "help" lines? We can also imagine the disappointment, and possible anger, she both felt for and anticipated receiving from her son. And we can understand how she might begin to suspect people in the local branch of the Credit Union of stealing from her; all that money gone and nothing to show for it. The disappointment and frustration, the overall emotional arousal of such an experience might give anyone high blood pressure. More significantly, these feelings might also introduce, if not reinforce, negative content in Merry's self-understanding with potential long-term negative consequences for her health.

I suggest that Merry's encounter with All Stars interacts with her experience of herself as an Aboriginal person. All Stars is a "big thing," a *munanga* thing, and the introduction of *munanga* into the scenario automatically entails the introduction of Aboriginal for the Aboriginal person schema arises from experiences of self in juxtaposition with or interacting with *munangas*. Here Merry is not simply a person, but an Aboriginal person, unable to achieve her goal derived from the *munanga* world. She may well experience herself as "hopeless" with not enough money to look after herself and her children, an experience that might parallel what is spoken of as "learned helplessness" (Seligman 1975) in some of the psychology literature.

Perhaps Merry sees herself not having enough money because she is an Aboriginal person and "Aboriginal people waste money," at least bad Aboriginal people who have not learned the "right way" do, to return to Lily's comments . Were Aboriginal person a relatively insignificant component of her self-understanding, Merry might never again experience herself as "hopeless," assuming she did on this occasion. But as I have argued, "Aboriginal person" is likely to be at the core of her identity. Not only is this likely to be an early lesson about self, Aboriginal people at Numbulwar interact with, or avoid, *munanga* and *munanga* things and *munanga* arrangements on a daily basis. If a great deal of Merry's experience with aspects of the *munanga* world has repeatedly led her to associate frustration of important goals with being an Aboriginal person, and if being an Aboriginal person is central to her self-understanding, then self becomes a threat to well-being insofar as a strong and automatic connection between self and frustration has been formed. Should this be the case for Merry, even when she is able to acquire or accomplish something she values as an Aboriginal person, self-experiences may include pain and frustration. Thus, experience of self has the potential to become a threat that is responded to by the fight-or-flight response (Brunner and Marmot 1999). Though I hope this is not the case, should Merry indeed be on her way to early illness and death, she is not alone on this journey.

Chapter 6

Selves and Others

Is it in the lineaments of our psychological natures that my flourishing as a member of my culture makes me less able to confront the challenges of a radically new future?

—Lear 2006:64

"Cultural Selves" and Others

Although she is speaking of Western Arrente "culture," the words of Austin-Broos (1996) seem to apply equally well to describe a contemporary Aboriginal identity, or more precisely to anticipate this chapter's focus, to facets of an Aboriginal self that may be widely shared at Numbulwar. It can be seen as "an extremely complicated one; both new and intractable, repositioned and yet unassimilated, dominated and yet recalcitrant." This complexity emerges as the "primordial" identity is engulfed by "an order of dominance bent on incorporation and production of 'ethnicity.'" Yet, "integral to this ethnicity are also dimensions of ontic experience from the past sustained unconsciously in the present" (5).

In the last chapter, I suggested that encounters such as Merry's with All Stars, especially when repeated many times, may lead to a sense of self characterized by excessively harmful feelings of pain and frustration, a posited source of premature morbidity and mortality. If we accept that these feelings arise when Aboriginal people engage with the *munanga* world, with the "new," "repositioned," and "dominated" sense of self, we might also ask where the "ontic experience from the past sustained unconsciously in the present"—the "intractable," the "unassimilated," the "recalcitrant" dimensions of Aboriginal identity—begins. This, perhaps not coincidentally, is just another version of the kinds of questions that whitefella missionaries, medical staff, and school teachers have been asking in a variety of ways over many years. Why have Aboriginal people changed so little, or changed in the ways that they have? Why, for example, are at least some members of the younger generations learning less rather than more English than their parents? Why does the school continue to be an institution that so many Aboriginal children avoid?

Psychological anthropologists have long attempted to understand the interactions of individual selves and their sociocultural settings. Drawing upon decades of culture-and-personality-inspired ethnography as well as upon contemporary efforts in neuroscience, Quinn (2003, 2005c) has reinvigorated these efforts with her analytic concept of a "cultural self." Early lessons about self that are accompanied by strong, but not overwhelming, emotion become core features of a species-specific brain as it emerges to become an individual mind of an individual self in a particular community. Insofar as the experiences of these lessons are shared—and much of this experience is shared, not only because of the shared characteristics of the learning minds but also because of the shared intentions of the enculturated teachers—we may speak of a cultural self. This is not to deny human individuality; the impossibility of identical experience is easily imagined of any learning situation. It is, however, a way to understand how people socialized in one cultural tradition rather than another may be more or less suited to one way of life rather than another.[1]

As Barry et al. (1959) believed they had discovered some years ago, a belief supported by a more recent study (Hendrix 1985), people try to socialize their children to become certain kinds of people, particularly people who do certain kinds of work. A shared model of socialization, as Quinn (2003:147) puts it, that "specifies the kind of adult child rearers desire to raise and a set of practices...thought to most effectively raise a child to be such an adult." Crucial here is her view that these lessons of early experience are enduring and highly motivating:they are instantiated in patterns of the brain's synapses that are "highly resolved," that is, they consist of "a pattern of synaptic firing in which the synapses involved are strongly connected to one another while not being connected, even weakly, to other synapses" (Quinn 2005c:480). To the extent that they arise from a culturally shared model of child socialization—a model that specifies both the kind of child to raise and how to do so—these lessons result in implicit cultural selves, selves that not only know what kind of people they are but selves that also want to be that kind of person.

The focal setting of this kind of early learning is, of course, the family. As I have mentioned in chapter four, this early learning is not only about self but also about others, and the first lessons are usually about those others we call family, regardless of the form that family might take. The associative nature of human learning (e.g., LeDoux 2002:134–70) suggests that as we internalize a culturally motivated model of self, so we are internalizing a culturally motivated model of others. Writing about an Aboriginal population in central Australia, Myers (1986) has cast the kind of familial sociality I speak of here as "autonomy" embedded in "relatedness" (109–11). When, as a part of the attachment process, children internalize what we may presume to be an experience of an "autonomous self"—the self that moves away from caretaker—so too do they internalize their experience of that "autonomous self" with "other"—the self that returns when feelings of separation anxiety compel it to do so. This, I believe , is the origin of relatedness. The feelings of security and anxiety that are an intrinsic part of the attachment cycle, and hence of this early experience, are repeatedly felt hundreds of times in our early years (Bowlby 1969) ensuring that an internalized model of others—a schema—is, like the self schema, enduring and motivational. The associative nature of human learning also suggests that our "self schema" will be strongly associated with our "others schema," or it might simply be best to speak of a "highly resolved" "self with others schema," at the core of which is our early experience of family.

Bedtime

The idea that the human mind "transfers meaning from that which is known...to that which otherwise must remain unknown and not understood" (Fernandez 1991:4) is both widespread and robust in terms of empirical support.[2] We might consider the possibility that the schema of "self with others" arising from early experiences of the "Aboriginal child with Aboriginal family" provides a template for experiencing Western institutions. We might also consider that in doing so this schema is the likely source of the "intractable," the "unassimilated," the "recalcitrant" dimensions of Aboriginal selves.

A contrast, however, must be drawn between the cultural models assumed by Quinn and Barry, et al., and those I posit for Numbulwar. Harmony between the "kind of adult child rearers desire to raise" and the kind of adult who "works" in the community appears to be characteristic of the former. In contrast, the cultural models motivating socialization at Numbulwar do not posit

an adult who works in either the Western sense or the Western setting. I remind readers that Numbulwar is an "intercultural" setting,
characterized by the divergence of blackfella and whitefella experience, not least because of what may be different value hierarchies
for each group. We find here "a line of development separate from
the [dominant] political and economic system of a society" (Kakar
1996:196).

Turning now to specifics, I illustrate the kinds of things Aboriginal
children in Numbulwar learn, or more precisely the kinds of things
they do not learn, using an example of early learning in middle-class
Anglo-American families. This learning accompanies what Shweder
et al. (1998) have called the institution of "bedtime" (873). The
practice associated with this institution is as follows. At a certain
time, specified by at least one parent, usually in the early evening,
children are told it is time for bed. When they are infants they are
simply placed in bed, sometimes in a room of their own, sometimes
with other children. Protests, crying, or saying "but I'm not sleepy"
are ultimately not effective ways of avoiding bedtime, though they
may be useful delaying tactics. The amount of space in parenting
manuals devoted to advice on how to get children to go to bed at
"bedtime" suggests the extent to which this practice often violates
what children really want to do.

Although my work does not include a systematic study of sleeping routines at Numbulwar, I say with some confidence, based on
my years of participant observation, that Western bedtime is not a
typical practice there. Children "go to bed" when adults do, or when
they just fall asleep. As Hamilton (1981) has observed of infants in
another remote Arnhem Land community:

> While European babies spend much of their time in cots and cribs,
> and even alone in a room with the door closed, Anbarra children are
> constantly exposed to all the sights and sounds of the camp...There
> are no routines of any kind to order this experience, other than the
> normal rhythms of the camp. (31–2)

On many occasions, as readers might have noted from interview
texts, I have asked of some act or another, "Why" (though the actual
phrasing in Aboriginal English is "What for") did somebody do
something. The following is from an interview I conducted in 2004
with Ngalba, an older woman first heard from in the last chapter.
The conversation is slightly unusual in my persistent questioning,
something I felt able to do with Ngalba and in her willingness to

express some exasperation with this interview technique:

> *VKB*: What for do some people have a no good life?
> *Ngalba*: Like they always get into trouble and have bad lives?
> *VKB*: Whatever you think. What for do some people get into trouble?
> *Ngalba*: Maybe they try to do good things, they try to have a good life but they make mistakes, they end up having a bad life.
> *VKB*: What for do they make mistakes?
> *Ngalba*: Maybe they can't think straight, they can't think properly what they are doing.
> *VKB*: What for can't they think properly?
> *Ngalba*: Maybe they like to do silly things, they like doing crazy things. Maybe you want to ask what for?
> *VKB*: Yes, I want to ask what for.
> *Ngalba*: Anthropologists are crazy.
> *VKB*: What for do they like doing silly things?
> *Ngalba*: They like doing it.

Ngalba's repeated refrain, "they like doing silly things," "they like doing crazy things," "they like doing it," is the kind of answer I have come to expect, a predictable response to my questions about why people do, or do not do, something. I believe that such phrases are not a way to end a conversation with an intrusive outsider, instead, they represent Aboriginal people's theory of motivation based on what they see going on around them and what they think about human nature. Indeed, Aboriginal people at Numbulwar do seem to do something and see themselves doing something because they "like doing it," just as they see themselves not doing something because they "don't like" doing it. The way one feels about doing something or not is a recognized and accepted motive. Children go to sleep when they feel sleepy, that is, "they like doing it."

Western Institutions

If local Aboriginal theory is precise in identifying "like doing" and "don't like doing" as core motivations, then it seems reasonable to posit these as components, indeed central components, of the cultural self. It is also easy to think these motivations character-istic of an "autonomous person." Hamilton (1981), however, has suggested that what varies in the early experiences of "European" and Anbarra children are the domains in which they are given or denied autonomy (148–53). This, I think, is a more accurate view. Doing what one likes doing is only a part of the picture. There are realms in which people cannot do what they like doing. These would include ritual, child-care, and, at least prior to settlement, kinship etiquette and marriage. These domains, however, have relatively little to offer as models for action within nonfamilial Western institutions. They are also domains that are, with the exception of some kinship etiquette, learned from late childhood on, a point whose importance will be seen in the discussion of children's experience of school.

I would describe "impersonality" as a focal characteristic of extra-familial Western institutions, for example, school and work, the institutions I am thinking of here. The personal has little place within them, and personal feelings are not recognized, at least as legitimate reasons for action. The contrast I have just drawn between personal and impersonal is perhaps the best evidence of this characteristic of Western culture, because persons, that is, people, are, of course, a part of institutions, which do not exist apart from them. However, the permissible aspects of people in institutions or people as institutions, apart from the institution of family, are parsed down to a very restricted version of what the person is. School and work are about doing a job, being on time, getting things done. At their core, they are not about how the people who function in them are feeling or getting on with their lives, though it must be said that in recent decades there has been some recognition of the personal (e.g., sick leave and maternity leave). It is still more likely, though, that if the personal interferes with getting the job done, something must be done about the person(al). It must be changed or people must leave.

It is, I think, this characteristic that repels many Aboriginal people, especially perhaps those from remote communities such as Numbulwar, when they want, or are required, to participate in Western institutions. School and work simply do not engage many of them because of the emotional incompatibility of the cultural self with a Western arrangement of others; thus the sense of senselessness when many Aboriginal people engage in Western acts. Rather than not seeing the point of doing something, they often do see the point. For example, one works in the shop to earn money to buy food. Critically, though, they do not feel the point. Hunting and fishing feel good because one engages in them when one feels like it, perhaps because one feels like eating a certain kind of food or sharing food with kin. Working in the shop may feel good one day, but not the next. Yet the job requires that one be there, whether one feels like it or not.

What is it about the Western experience that contributes to a cultural self that, at least for many, perhaps especially from the middle classes, enables participation in extra-familiar institutions? Presumably, Western children, just like Aboriginal children, entering impersonal institutions for the first time "transfer... meaning from that which is known" (Fernandez 1991:4), that is, they initially use the self with other (as family) schema to understand self with other as, say, school experience. Yet for many Western children there may be much less dissonance with which to contend. The answer to this question may be that many Western families, particularly those that produce children who "fit in," incorporate into the cultural self a sense of the impersonal. Bedtime is not the only early experience of the schedule that many Western children have. Even in households where "schedule feeding" is no longer the norm, where "mealtime" is no longer an occasion, there are likely to be adults and siblings who routinely have to be somewhere or do something "on time." Schedules as used in the West are impersonal. They are fixed by convention and are not usually to be varied according to how one feels.

Family Again

As foreshadowed earlier, the "kind of adult child rearers desire to raise" (Quinn 2003:142) seems to be premised on shared understandings of the kind of adult who "works" in the community (Barry et al. 1959; Hendrix 1985). Socialization anticipates a particular kind of cultural self that fits in with a particular kind of cultural others whom we may expect to be moral others.

From the perspective of cognitive linguistics, Lakoff and Johnson (1999) understand metaphor as a form of thought arising from experiences of our bodies interacting with our world (45–9). The understandings that emerge from these concrete, first-order experiences, such as object manipulation or standing upright, enable and permeate more abstract thought. Thus, for example, our understandings of time, mind, and self are essentially metaphorical. To say that much of our thought is metaphorical, however, is not to dismiss its utility; to the extent that a metaphor is apt, it enables learning, understanding, and functioning. Morality is also experienced and understood via metaphors that arise from bodily experience, particularly that of "ill"- or "well-being" (290). Metaphors that underlie the expression of various moral ideas arise in universal human experiences of what is good and bad for people. That is, such conditions as health, strength, resources (wealth), autonomy, social capital, and nurturance are usually seen as good for people, while their opposites, such as illness, weakness, poverty, constraint, social isolation, and neglect, are usually seen as bad for people (see also Nussbaum 1995). It is from such experiences as these that we develop ideas about what should and should not be done to people, including our self.

According to Lakoff and Johnson (1999), these experiences and associated metaphors are various and not necessarily compatible. The coherence we find in moral systems is provided by models of the family; that is, our folk model (or models) of the family "organizes our overall moral outlook" (334). If Lakoff and Johnson are right, then family does not simply provide an enduring and motivating schema of self with others, it also provides a metaphor of morality and our sense of morality, of what is good and bad, grounds our hierarchy of values and moves us to action (Elzanowski 1993). Thus, I expect a schema of self with others as family to be a primary motivating force, at the core of a cultural self.[3]

What model, or models, of the family might be employed at Numbulwar? Lakoff and Johnson (1999) offer an array of possibilities positioned between two somewhat polarized ideal types of family model, the "strict father" (which may be a "strict mother") and the "nurturing parent," though they emphasize that most models are either variants or blends of the two (311–18). Elements of both these models capture what may be the experience of family in Numbulwar: fathers may be seen as "strict," insofar as they do have power over the child and may teach by moral example; both mothers and fathers may nurture and protect the child. Family life is more variable and complex than this, however, and the child's experience and resulting schema can also be expected to be more varied and more complex.

Since settlement, whether at the Roper River, Groote Eylandt, or Rose River Mission, major changes in family structure and function have taken place. As we saw in chapter three, marriage has shifted from polygyny to monogamy. Increasingly young women's, indeed teenagers', first experience of parenthood is as a single parent (Burbank 1988; Burbank and Chisholm 1998). Divorce is not uncommon, and mothers and fathers sometimes move away both from the community and from their children. And while it has undoubtedly always been the case that parents of young children die, this may now be a more common occurrence. The extended family continues to predominate, both in terms of residence in the same house or in a group of neighboring houses and in terms of function. Sometimes, one's mother, say, may live in another part of town but no house on the settlement is located beyond easy walking distance and many daily routines include visiting family who live in other parts of town . Children and adults move back and forth between related households for a variety of reasons, both practical and social. Mothers' brothers and fathers' sisters continue to be given parental-type authority over their siblings' offspring, and grandparents are often primary carers, if only by default. Older siblings and cousins, both male and female, may also, from time to time nurture, protect and "boss" younger children. The diverse combinations of residence and care undoubtedly provide a variety of family experience.

The Equivalence of Family Members

There is one characteristic, however, that I believe is a part of any child's family schema. This can be labeled the "principle of the equivalence of family members."

Anthropologists describing kinship in Aboriginal Australia have long made reference in their accounts to the "principle of the equivalence of same-sex siblings" (e.g., Berndt and Berndt 1964; Tonkinson 1978:43). That is, if one knows the term one calls, say, a woman, one knows that one calls all her actual sisters by that same term; and, all things being equal (though they often are not), one knows that one calls her classificatory sisters by the same term as well. Equivalence as a principle of family is more pervasive than this, however. Let us begin, as Scheffler (1978) might suggest we do, though our intent is not an analysis of kinship per se, with the Aboriginal theory of parent/child links at Numbulwar. As a general rule, children are said to "come from" their father and their father's country, and are thus entitled to share his country and clan and by extension, moiety. That is, the child is the "same" as the father with regard to country, clan, and moiety identity. Children are the totemic creatures of their father's country, just as are their fathers. Meeting a stranger, either father or child might say, for example, "I am emu." In dreams, children are represented by their mother's image or totems. A dream about a woman or any of her Dreaming animals presages the arrival of her child, who calls her totems "milk," that is, mother. Fathers

give children their face and their feet, "just like father"; both mothers and fathers sustain children with their bodies. When the child
is a fetus, both mother and father grow thin before they grow fat.
After birth, as the child grows, mother and father weaken:

> The child takes mother's and father's body and makes them weak.
> Like [a man and his wife]. They are strong because they don't have
> any children. They are a bit old but still strong, not like [the man's
> brother] who has children. He is weak. (Aboriginal woman in
> Burbank 1980:47)

In a manner not unlike Sökefeld's self (1999) discussed in chapter
five, the fetus acts as a homunculus with regard to maternal feelings
and actions:

> Maybe that girl is gonna be pregnant and that baby is gonna tempt
> her mother, that girl is gonna make fights all the time because she is
> starting to have that baby...old people can tell that way when they
> fight, that means they gonna have a baby...She is gonna be jealous
> all the time. (Aboriginal woman in Burbank 1994:60)

In chapter two we saw that the equivalence of family members is
such that the transgression of one may lead to the punishment unto
death of all. We also saw, in chapter four, the extension of this belief
in sorcery accounts where it is said that if a sorcerer cannot kill
his intended victim, he may be satisfied by killing another family
member.

The relationship of equivalence is simultaneously a relationship
of reciprocity and so we may say that a moral principle of reciprocity and its negative forms of revenge and retribution accompany the
principle of equivalence in the family schema. According to Lakoff
and Johnson (1999) who posit these moral substitutes, reciprocity,
revenge and retribution as moral ideas derive from the observation
that well-being is a limited resource that can be augmented or diminished by the actions of others (293–8). A moral act is thus one where
the well-being of another is increased. A moral act, however, may
also be a reciprocal act affecting well-being, whether for ill or good.
Use of "square back," a term for something one can do in return for
an act of sharing or an act of aggression, suggests the psychological
validity (Wallace 1961) of this idea in the community.

Reciprocity between children and parents begins during pregnancy. Pregnant women should eat lots of fish, turtle, and dugong
to make the baby fat. The baby in turn makes both its mother and

father *walaj*, good or successful hunters. When women notice another catching a great deal of fish, they may suspect a pregnancy, "Might be that baby is helping his mommy" (Burbank 1980:47). Later, women, at least in past times, would help a son by not eating:

> Emu and bush turkey have strong power. If you eat them and somebody is fighting, the spear will come to you. They make you deaf and you fight. Younger boys can eat and women can always eat, but when a man is young neither he nor his mother will eat things like emu, turkey or fat from dugong and turtle...If he does eat emu, when somebody throws a spear he won't run away. He will throw back and kill that man...The women do this because this is the Law; they help the boy. If a boy eats, he will be cranky and fighting. If his mother eats, she won't get cranky, but he will. (Aboriginal woman in Burbank 1999:45)

Fights, which have been common events at Numbulwar during my various visits, are always occasions for reciprocity. Among other kin, mothers, mothers' brothers, fathers, fathers' sisters, and, conversely, adult children "take partner" or act as *wajar* (a protective referee-like role) for one another. These are especially telling examples, for fights in this community are often moral family dramas (cf. MacDonald 1988). A single fight may represent immorality in the violation of Law; the assertion of morality via the punishment of the wrongdoer; and nurturing, the intervention of people in a parenting role who may even refer to their intervention as "minding," as in "I'm minding all those kids" (Burbank 1994:76). Reciprocity—that is, assisting a family member—revenge and retribution are also typical aspects of fights:

> [Those mothers of the boys and their sister] should be here looking after their husbands and sons. Their sons almost killed each other. And those three are off acting like young girls. When they come back I am going to ask [a woman] for six eggs. I'll tell her I'm hungry, but that's only gammon [a lie]. I'll throw two at [the mother's sister], two for [one mother], and two for [the other mother]. If that old man had died, I would cut off all three of their heads with a galiwanga [a large knife]. I have a long one there at the house. I don't want any *wajar* [intervention], nobody be *wajar* for me. Poor [youth who shot the gun]. They took him off to jail. (Aboriginal woman in Burbank 1994:76)

Thus, whatever else may be in the family schema of people in the community, it is highly likely that it includes a principle of the equivalence of family members and a moral valence that is expressed in ideas about reciprocity, revenge, and retribution.

It is also clear that feelings are an inextricable part of the schema. As Quinn (2003) observes, early socialization almost invariably includes some degree of emotional arousal, through the inducement of physical and/or psychic pleasure or pain via techniques such as praising, teasing, and frightening. The presence of emotion at a time of learning has the effect of consolidating that learning.[4] Again, because learning is associational, the emotions associated with the experience of that learning come to be associated with the lessons that are learned. For example, if shaming is the means by which a lesson about self is conveyed to the child, a feeling of shame is associated with the aspect of self the child has learned by being shamed (148–9; 2005c: 491–9). I once asked a woman if "feeling family," words used by another women, meant that family members know how others in the family are feeling. She replied, "We think we know how they are feeling, but we don't know. We watch how they act if they are upset." In fact, the routine practice of asking children what they want to do, rather than assigning them to a setting or activity against their will, indicates that others do not expect to know how family members feel. People do see family members as the cause of feelings, though. The embryo "tempts" mother's jealousy. A mother's diet produces aggression in her son and, as proposed in chapter four, "family" can make people feel good and/or bad. In the following text, family determines the well- or ill-being of both children and adults. As Ngalba, speaking here, presents it, family has the power to "upset," to give or withhold "hope." Not only does a parent's separation take away hope from a child, but also having one's own family and caring for them gives or evokes happiness in the adult. The connection between emotions and family is also presented here within a reciprocal, or even retributive, framework:

> VKB: You say some young people got no hope, some young people got hope. What makes them different?
>
> Ngalba: Some got hope. They find a job and that makes them feel good, they earn money and they understand how to take care of themselves. Maybe another young person thinks he doesn't got no hope from his parents, their parents are separated. They get upset, so do silly things, get upset, think that's the only way, upset himself and his family, go to jail. But he's got hope, to live. If he tries to do them wrong things, still he's got the hope to live and he realises maybe thinking, "I gotta stop doing this." They get upset because they haven't got any family around and go do silly thing

to ruin themself. But, there are people, he's got someone there to help him, to talk to him to leave that sort of a thing, people who love him. He can change from doing that rubbish thing to leading a good life. And that somebody, whoever, he's happy with his job, with what he's doing, he feels good, he's got a job, he's got money. Maybe [his] family too, got family, you know, to support them and take care of them kids and feel happy maybe to his family, helping them. (Ngalba 2003)

Going to School and Work

Turning away from family at Numbulwar to its Western institutions, we see that the first such institution with which most Aboriginal people are likely to have sustained contact is the school. Peopled by what I see as a dedicated staff, both Aboriginal and non-Aboriginal, the school is, nevertheless, at its foundation, an impersonal institution. This impersonality is highlighted by the 2002 Northern Territory Curriculum Framework (NTCF) and the associated "process of substantially implementing an outcome-focused approach to planning, teaching-learning, and assessment and reporting" (iii). The concept of "outcome" enables us to see that, like so many other institutions of learning today, the metaphor used not only to describe but also to prescribe, and thus construct, the reality of the school is that of a business with a product, that is, an "outcome." Whether expressed as outcome or product, businesses produce things.[5] They are not there, according to the business metaphor, to nurture people. In transferring meaning from the known to the unknown, the likely schema of self with other that Aboriginal children project onto the school is far from impersonal. It includes a self that is autonomous with regard to domains associated with body rhythms and daily routines, in contrast to schedules, which are the epitome of the impersonal. The school is run on schedule with set times to begin and end, some signaled, as mentioned in chapter two, by a recorded ringing bell or piano music: "time to" do certain kinds of lessons, "time to" engage in certain activities.

The child's schema is also likely to include a principle of the equivalence of family members and a moral valence expressed in ideas about reciprocity, revenge, and retribution, including reciprocity of feeling, whether this leads to negative or positive interaction. Here, the school may be more schema friendly, so to speak. As we have seen, whitefella teachers are incorporated into the kinship system, and they often appear to act as would kin toward the schoolchildren.

Aboriginal adults also have a notable presence at the school, and some children are likely to have a close relative present in class or nearby. The Aboriginal teachers, instructors in the language revitalization program and assistant teachers do, sometimes, act as kin. For example, when a post-primary girl was "teasing"[6] another girl, an assistant teacher and "close family" member of the victim "took partner" and struck the aggressor. Sometimes, their presence as kin disrupts the schedule, as when another assistant teacher spent the first five minutes or so of a post-primary class talking about a fight in the community that had occurred the previous day. Many mothers, grandmothers, or other female relatives of schoolchildren wait in the school yard during class time, meeting the children at the 11:00 break, often providing them with food or with money to buy food from the tuck shop. However, many children do not have an adult relative in class, and, at school, whitefella teachers do not, indeed cannot, really act as kin. Nor can the Aboriginal teachers, language instructors, and assistant teachers often act as kin to their kin, because they are usually acting as expected in their school role.

It is important to remember that schemas are not fixed. In the process of enabling understanding, they do not block new information, but are the means by which new information and understanding are acquired (D'Andrade 1995:141–9; Strauss and Quinn 1997:98–101). Schoolchildren can come to understand school as a place where the self is not autonomous with regard to what they are going to do at a certain time. They can also come to understand that school is a place where kin cannot always act as kin. We must keep in mind, however, the motivational force of the early schema, which comes from the feelings associated with it. For the Aboriginal child, or so I argue here, these are largely such feelings as "like doing" and "feeling family." These are also largely, I think, good feelings in so far as schemas include feelings associated with their acquisition. Thus, when there is competition for the schoolchild's time and attention, when family matters arise, as they often do, school is easy to give up. That is to say, school is not the only game in town; and family feels better.[7]

Not going to school, or work, is not necessarily a univalent experience, however. It feels good, or so I argue here, but it may also feel bad. Over the years, for example, school personnel have worked hard to encourage school attendance. The "Two-Way Learning" program that incorporates some aspects of local culture into school practice received major impetus during the years when the local Aboriginal woman was principal. Although she no longer resides in the community, much of her effort has been maintained by the staff, and the school regularly holds "culture days" with "traditional" dancing and barbecues. Local people are invited to speak to children about past practices, for example, mother-in-law bestowal, and their talks are recorded and incorporated into lessons aimed at language renewal or English literacy. Prizes, such as bicycles and footballs, are awarded at school assemblies for various accomplishments. Children are taken on both local and distant field trips. In 2004, the school held a three-day "Woman's Camp," and then a three-day "Men's Camp," at a distant coastal outstation, where days were spent in fishing and hunting and evenings in various educational and recreational activities. In 2005, a post-primary teacher bleached the hair of those who had attended school five days in a row, for a look that many teenagers seem to desire. So the school schema may also have positive values and feelings associated with it. The child who does not go to school misses out on desirable acquisitions and activities that are fun.

Although, at least for some children, both school and family are associated with positive feelings, when both are juxtaposed in circumstances that may be described as competitive, the family schema may dominate because it is such an emotional schema and is more motivating than that of school. In such circumstances, the subjective experience may be a dissonant one, one of comfort, of feeling "like doing" and "feeling family" and, simultaneously, one of anger, disappointment, or boredom, feelings that further motivate a withdrawal, whether psychic or physical, from the activity at hand. Thus, the acculturating process is resisted but, as always, there are costs to this resistance. Withdrawal from the Western institution in which participation was initially desired may be accompanied by other feelings, such as alienation and hopelessness, feelings that then, because they are associated with both family and school, become as much a part of the family schema as that of the Western institution.

Interacting with Whitefellas

There is more, however, to the "extremely complicated" cultural self, providing, as it may, representations of "experience from the past sustained unconsciously in the present" yet required to interact with an "order of dominance bent on incorporation (Austin-Broos 1996:5)".

I suggested in chapter two that the "adoption" of whitefellas into Aboriginal family was more of a social necessity for Aboriginal people than might first be apparent. If this is indeed the case, the practice, in all likelihood, is motivated by a "cultural self." I have also proposed that early experiences of family provide an enduring and motivating schema of self with others and a sense of morality that grounds a hierarchy of values. It is within a context created by such a self, morality, and value hierarchy that blackfellas and *munangas* try to interact.

If we accept that the whitefellas and blackfellas of Numbulwar are guided by separate hierarchies of value that may be distinguished more by the way they give precedence to values when they come into conflict than in the content of the values themselves, it seems clear that for Aboriginal people, relationships, especially those with family, generally take precedence over most if not all Western institutions and arrangements. It also seems clear that relationships take precedence over things. While I can't say that whitefellas always value material success above their relationships with others, there are more occasions, and arrangements, where we can see just such precedence being given to the impersonal, "things" in the Western context; sometimes other considerations take precedence over relationships, and smooth relations, with their fictive Aboriginal kin. Here, for example, is an account of just such a case that I obtained from a whitefella:

> NUD: [An Aboriginal woman] used to work at [a job] and drive the Troopy [from troop-carrier, a four wheel drive vehicle]. She got [her son] to drive the Troopy because she was getting in and out and taking things to people all the time. He didn't have a license and was using the vehicle to go to the airstrip. Someone at the office questioned him and he went off his head and drove the Troopy 120 K [per hour] around town—it's lucky no one was killed—and deliberately tried to smash it against poles and damaged it and it couldn't be driven until we spent about $10,000 to fix it.
>
> VKB: $10,000!
>
> NUD: Well, it cost $40,000. We were told...we shouldn't have done that, questioned him. (NUD 2003)

The following interpretation of whitefella and blackfella actions that I obtained from an Aboriginal woman Sunny (2003) appears to focus on the same event; it was one that many were talking about at the time of both interviews: "White people go angry. Because some Aboriginal people driving Council vehicle don't got license. They go fast. They can't see that sign for 40 or 60 [kilometers per hour].

[Then] Aboriginal people go angry to *munanga*."[8] When Aboriginal people drive Council vehicles without a license and drive over the speed limit, whitefellas get angry at them. In response, Aboriginal people get "angry" back at them.

Respective blackfella, whitefella value hierarchies and the way they may come into conflict are manifest in this incident if indeed Sunny and the whitefella are speaking of the same event. Actions that a whitefella described as questioning were interpreted by Sunny as an expression of anger. According to her text, the young man interpreted the whitefella questioning as such and matched white-fella anger with his own. This young man appears to have been giving priority, first of all, to his mother's needs. In doing so he violated the whitefella rules and procedures of primary value to them. Subsequently, he gave priority to the expression of his anger, provoked, perhaps, by the challenge to his autonomy that question-ing represented. Although he might have endangered some as an unintended consequence of his mad drive though the town, he did not attack the people who "questioned him," even verbally as far as I know. This suggests that even in his anger he held people, relation-ships, and their well-being in higher regard than he did the physi-cal condition of a vehicle. However, he damaged the costly vehicle, highly valued by the whitefellas.

Many, if not the majority of whitefellas at Numbulwar appeared to engage with Aboriginal people in genuine and positive ways. Some whitefellas, for example, went fishing with Aboriginal friends; some invited Aboriginal people to join them for meals and responded with generosity to requests for money and other items or assistance. I always saw whitefellas at all the funerals I attended. School teach-ers, in particular, attended the *wunubal* at the deceased's house on days prior to a funeral; they made concerted efforts to attend the public parts of circumcision ceremonies and, as mentioned earlier, supported the teaching of Wubuy and a fortnightly "culture day" of Aboriginal music and dancing at the school. These acts seemed to take place in an environment of mutuality. Aboriginal people made sure that whitefellas knew they were welcome at such ceremonies, brought them portions of their hunting and fishing catches and pre-sented them with gifts of baskets, paintings, and carvings that they or their kin had made.[9]

Such positive forms of attention from whitefellas is something that makes at least some Aboriginal people feel good. Here, for example, Gerard (2003), the twenty-eight-year-old father of two, who tells a story about positive interaction with a whitefella in chapter five, talks about his experiences in Darwin, where the band he plays with went on tour:

> Last year or this year, July, I went for that [tour]. I went...to play concert at Darwin, dancing concert. And that funeral at Bagot [an Aboriginal settlement in the Darwin area]...Like whitefellas come to us and...write our name in the paper. And they said, "This the first time Aborigine went to dance culture"...We went to one place in Darwin, Mindil Beach and we did lots of dancing, performing there, showing some white people. Make me feel good.

Gerard and the rest of the band took part in a concert, played for a funeral in an Aboriginal community close to Darwin and performed at Mindil Beach, an open air market listed as one of Darwin's tourist attractions. When I asked if any good things happened during the tour, Gerard told about the journalist writing it up. Performing for whitefellas, "showing some" people the dances, made Gerard "feel good." Whitefellas may not, however, always be attentive to black-fella needs, even those who are "kin." Here, Gerard speaks about asking a whitefella to fix his washing machine:

> Like some white people, some white people a bit angry, taking over, come here don't like Aboriginal people. When we tell white people to do something, nothing. Like maybe we go and tell whitefella here, I went to tell him to fix my washing machine. He was a bit angry at me but I didn't bother.

Nor may whitefella kin be as accessible as other kin. For example, the majority of whitefellas that I asked said they discouraged children from visiting and others said they had little to do with Aboriginal people outside their working roles: "We don't really mix with them; [our job] is all we can handle. We're tired at the end of the day" (STL 2005). One or two of the whitefellas appeared to be at Numbulwar to stay, as in the case of the widower mentioned by Vikki in chapter five. Most whitefellas, however, are people who leave:

> VKB: How long do you think you'll stay?
> NUD: I'll probably stay another year. The job is really good. But I want to see a difference, I want to see self-determination really happen. After a while you need job satisfaction, seeing that you are accomplishing something. I enjoy my job, it's the context that's [so hopeless]. After a while you think, "What's the point?" (NUD 2003)

When Numbulwar was Rose River Mission, at least some of the whitefellas stayed for long periods of time. Recall, from chapter two, that the Reverend Earl Hughes worked there for at least seventeen years. One nursing sister that I met on my first trip to Numbulwar was, during this last series of visits, still fondly recalled. She had, I believe, served as a missionary-nurse for close to twenty years. Those days may be over, however. On all of my trips to Numbulwar, I have invariably found that whitefellas from previous visits have moved on. Aboriginal people are accustomed to losing their whitefella kin. Some may even grieve for their loss (cf. Austin-Broos 2009:130).

Orphans

At least since the Whitlam Labour Government of the early 1970s, Australian government policy has largely manifested at Numbulwar in increasing, though by Western standards inadequate, amounts of material infrastructure and consumer goods. When Kinsey tells us, as she did in chapter five, that "if you want to make yourself *munanga*, you want to buy everything," especially "big" whitefella things, she puts her finger on what I see as the resounding significance of whitefellas in Aboriginal lives, at least in recent years. Whitefellas are people who both possess highly desirable items and mediate, whether directly or indirectly, Aboriginal possibilities to also possess them. I doubt that my currency at Numbulwar (an interesting metaphor in light of this discussion) has ever been so high as it was in 1978 when the "grant" I wrote for a "landrover," among other items for a planned outstation, was successful; Sherry clearly sees this mediation when she says that Aboriginal people "want education, they want to learn more. And then they grow up they work to school, office, respite, homeland."

Aboriginal people without whitefellas things, such as money and mobile phones, are sometimes described as *wangulu*, "orphans," though the people so described are as inextricably intermeshed with family as are the speakers. From my perspective, there are "real" orphans at Numbulwar, that is, children without parents; and though they may not fare quite as well as children with living parents, they do have family. What being a *wangulu* seems to really mean is that someone has no one to look after them. Here, for example, is an exchange with Merry (2005) when I asked for the translation of "orphan":

Merry: Like I pick Spike and Jay, got no mother. Their mother pass away, but they get support from me and [their father's brother].

Even his [the two boys] father too, cause he got no wife. [We support these two boys and their father].
VKB: How do I say this in Kriol?
Merry: *Wangulu.* They are really not *wangulu.* They get support from me.
VKB: So if no support, that's *wangulu*?
Merry: Proper true *wangulu.*

Merry is saying that orphans are people without "support" whether or not they have parents. If Merry did not support him, a man without a wife could be regarded as a *wangulu*. People who leave Numbulwar, and family, to go "touristing" in Darwin, "sleep in the long grass, *wangulu* people." Or "When you go anywhere and ask anyone for money and they can't give you, they say *wangulu*" (Sherry 2005). Why are people without things, or people to whom others don't wish to give things, being called orphans? The Pintupi word for orphan is *yapunta*, which is also used to signify that an object "does not belong to anyone" but might also "mean that it has no one holding or looking after it" (Myers 1988:55). If we follow Myers' lead in viewing objects as signifiers of autonomy and relatedness among Aboriginal people, we are directed to look again at "demand sharing," this time in order to understand how not having things and orphans are connected in the minds of at least some people. Recall, from chapter four, that demand sharing may be understood as a mechanism for the production and maintenance of relationships (Peterson 1993). When someone asks for something, they may indeed wish to have it, but more significantly, they may be testing, maintaining, or creating a relationship; withholding something that someone asks for in these circumstances risks being seen as the repudiation of a relationship.

If people regarded as kin never, or rarely, share, their lack of generosity may be interpreted as a lack of feeling for the other, a devaluation of the relationship or even dislike and repudiation of their kin (Myers 1986:115). However, reading Myers, Peterson (1993) suggests that not giving may sometimes be construed as an expression of autonomy rather than a lack of feeling . Such might be the interpretation if the person who withholds something has in the past been generous (868).[10] Whitefellas, however, even though they may be family, are strange kin indeed; they do not generally have extended histories of close, mutual relationships with their Aboriginal family. Consequently, when they do not share it may be all too easy for Aboriginal people to interpret this as a repudiation of their bond.

The question that we now need to ask is if people without mobile phones see themselves as abandoned by the encompassing society, a kind of family represented by their whitefella kin. We also need to ask, less rhetorically, perhaps, what can a *wangulu* do in such circumstances?

Throughout this work, the version of schema theory provided by Strauss and Quinn has enabled me to understand cultural and intercultural processes; it has also provided me with a way of understanding how human minds are able to assimilate new experience via the existing schema of past experience. However, this potential to act in unfamiliar circumstances does not imply that our improvised action is necessarily optimal action, nor may our emerging schema advance our fortunes in new situations. The utility of our improvisation, including satisfaction of our needs and with our selves, may require information about the new circumstance we simply do not have. It may also require us to be something we simply are not, nor want to be. Those of us with marginalized identities are as likely to value who we are as those of us whose are not so marginalized (Agar and Reisinger 2001:738).

Just as "whitefellas" have likely become a part of an Aboriginal family schema, so too might they be a part of an Aboriginal "self" schema. It is their very presence that leads to that facet of an Aboriginal self that we label "Aboriginal identity." This component may well include knowledge of how to get and keep whitefella things. However, having a "strong *binji*"—the ability to refuse requests and not share—among other necessary *munanga* capabilities may require years of training and practice that most Aboriginal people at Numbulwar never get. More critically a strong *binji* may also be experienced as a "not me" part of the self, something an Aboriginal person may both consciously and unconsciously refuse. Whitefellas, though they often come in handy and may be genuinely valued in some respects, are not, perhaps for many, people to emulate, except in superficial ways.

On my last visit to Numbulwar in 2007, I should not have been too surprised to hear of "Satan" making an appearance in accounts of black magic, piloting a plane that brings people of evil intent to the town . After all, the devil-beliefs of Columbian peasants and Bolivian miners have been interpreted as a response to an "evil and destructive" capitalist mode of production that increasingly penetrates their way of life (Taussig 1980:17). Surely something similar might be said of Numbulwar. The idea of Satan, of course, is derived from Christianity, which, though now largely in the hands of Aboriginal people, often seems to tell its adherents to turn their backs on "culture." Is giving up culture, and not simply perhaps an Aboriginal identity, but one's very, and, of course, cultural, self seen as the price one must pay to be included in the larger, increasingly desirable and increasingly necessary, sociality? If this is the case, then we might understand accounts of "black magic" not simply as a means of responding to death and loss, but also as a means of responding to what may be even more threatening experiences. We might imagine that talk of black magic speaks to feelings that arise from experiences of being excluded by the larger, predominantly whitefella society: feelings of frustration that accompany attempts to achieve *munanga* things, whether material or social, and feelings of abandonment, of whitefella family abandoning self or, for at least a few, of self abandoning Aboriginal family. Are these the kinds of feelings that are implicated in the genesis of premature disability, illness, and death?[12]

Chapter 7

Conclusion: A Tentative Answer to a Fundamental Epidemiological Question

A Fundamental Epidemiological Question

This ethnography of stress has now reached a place where I can provide a tentative answer to what Agar (2003) describes as a "fundamental epidemiological question—why these people in this place at this time?" (3). This is clearly a question that the disproportionate incidence of premature morbidity and mortality in Aboriginal Australia invites us to ask. As is the case with heroin addiction in American inner cities, premature death "is never randomly distributed. It always clusters among some social types and not among others." Agar directs us to look at "relevant systems" and "major ongoing changes" associated with "the social cluster within which incidence is on the rise" (3–4). I agree with him, and with Bourgois (2003), who says that "the larger historical structural forces that create vulnerable social groups" (26)—what Farmer (2004) calls "structural violence"—are essential components of such an account. I trust this is apparent in what I have presented in the preceding chapters. My answer, however, focuses primarily on "a kind of consciousness brought about by a kind of history" (Agar 2003:26), though I have argued that this "kind of consciousness" is, in fact, largely unconscious.

A Tentative Answer

The Aboriginal people of Numbulwar bear a legacy of extreme, by which I mean unhealthy, stress that likely goes back for over a century. This legacy may have begun in the late 1800s, either via direct experiences or from frightening accounts of disruption and brutality that accompanied the movement of colonial Australians into the north of the continent. The protection that Aboriginal people received from the missions and welfare bodies of the Federal and Territory governments had their costs, not simply in the disruption of a hunting and gathering way of life but also in the accompanying loss of autonomy and control. This kind of loss has characterized the lives of Aboriginal people at Numbulwar ever since.

In the social determinants of health literature, loss of autonomy and control, in particular, is associated with the kinds of afflictions that the Aboriginal people of Numbulwar, along with Aboriginal people across the continent, suffer from today: high blood pressure, obesity, diabetes, coronary heart disease, kidney failure, and depression. Inadequate and unsanitary housing, abuse of tobacco, cannabis, and alcohol, poor diet, and lack of exercise do not support human health. Nor do decayed teeth and lack of dental care, overcrowding, and repeated exposure to the kinds of violence that seem to have made an appearance at Numbulwar in recent years.[1] The social determinants literature, however, suggests that even without these health perturbations, these subordinated and disadvantaged people would fall ill and die in greater numbers at earlier ages than people in more advantaged populations, people like many, if not most, non-Indigenous Australians.

One source of this ill health may be located in the experiences of past generations. According to the fetal origins view of disease, an individual's fragility may originate not simply with a mother's or a mother's mother's stress, but with the stress of a pregnant woman from times long past (Kuzawa 2005). A woman whose pregnancy is punctuated by episodes of hunger, social disruption, anger, and fear is likely to be less able to adequately nourish her developing fetus, not simply because she does not have enough to eat, but because stress has the capacity to interfere with many physiological processes, including those of gestation. Whether the children born of such a woman are female or male, they, in turn, may be less able to care for their own offspring; their parenting capacities may have been compromised by their own fetal origins. A female's physiology may be one less able to sustain a healthy pregnancy and hence a healthy child; a male might also have frailties that diminish his parenting abilities, whether physical or psychological. In circumstances where the sources of such harmful stress have been widespread, even a man not adversely affected by his fetal origins might marry, reproduce, and parent with a woman who had been so affected.

As the fetal origins literature makes clear, however, an initial vulnerability does not invariably lead to premature morbidity and mortality. These consequences depend on the interaction of prenatal vulnerabilities with the postnatal environment.[2] There are, no doubt, many reasonably healthy people in the world whose minds and bodies bear some sort of frailty of prenatal origin. It is likely, however, that such people live in an environment characterized by relative comfort, both physical and psychological, and relative plenty, both material and social. In contrast, an environment characterized by poverty and social disadvantage is one designed to injure the health of anyone whatever their fetal origins. I have presented the environment of Numbulwar as a kind of intercultural creation with considerable potential to do such damage, not least because of the affective and moral disjunctions between "family" and extra-familial Western institutions. This potential may be more assisted than ameliorated by that facet of self we call an "Aboriginal" identity. I am not saying that everything about this environment is bad for people's health, nor that Aboriginal identity is a source only of bad feelings and stress. There are aspects of life at Numbulwar that undoubtedly nourish and support its residents. One that I have discussed is family, though discussions in chapters four and six make it clear that family is a social arrangement not without complications; it would seem to be the locus, of "complex and dynamic links" in Aboriginal lives. Being an "Aboriginal person" is a source of pride, at least for some. However, as the discussion in chapter five suggests, the experience of an Aboriginal identity is not a unidirectional one with a single, and positive, valence; in and of itself it may be a major source of "harmful, threatening or challenging conditions."

If we see the development of foundational schemas of self with others arising from the interaction of our species specific human potentials and deliberate, culturally grounded attempts to socialize children to live with others in specific ways, we can understand the observation that although "the interrelations between [autonomy and relatedness] appear to be a basic human phenomenon," "the particular ways these relations play out are different in different cultures" (Fajans 2006:190). We find specific, not generic schemas of self with others.[3] It is in the specificity of these schemas, especially in the ways they may differ between communities, that we find the basis for Aboriginal and whitefella experience of self with others, and their respective cultural selves. It is also in these specificities that I locate the difficulties that Aboriginal people have with themselves; the core of a cultural self provides both the best and the worst for the Aboriginal people of Numbulwar. It enables them to derive satisfaction and comfort from their family circumstances while it prevents them from engaging in the kinds of activities required for a satisfying and comfortable integration into the larger society. It is apparent that the people of Numbulwar have never been provided with genuine opportunity or with an adequate preparation for such integration, but it is also apparent that such integration would require many, if not most, to abandon their selves in ways unacceptable to them. The refusal to do so, seen on a daily basis in the actions of people I know, speaks to the repulsion with which this possibility is met. Unfortunately, while the impersonality of white-fella institutions and arrangements renders them unattractive, for the most part, whitefella things, particularly material things, hold great appeal. However, a cultural self ill suited to whitefella society makes whitefella things hard to come by. The experiences associated with the relative poverty and social disadvantage that this entails, the frustrations associated with being an Aboriginal person, under-mine satisfaction and comfort in the family, generate social trauma, perpetuate dysfunction, and exacerbate the likelihood of early ill-ness and death.

Necessary Sociality

My approach in this book has been oriented by the certainty that humans are of necessity social creatures and as such must pay atten-tion to others. We seem to accomplish this via our feelings (e.g., Fessler and Haley 2003; Reddy 2001:25) and increasingly we see evidence that "overlapping neural processes" are involved in experiences of both physical and social pain—that is, the "pain" of social exclu-sion (Eisenberger and Lieberman 2004). This possibility speaks to the harm that may be done by a variety of social experiences such as those we might call "discrimination," "marginalization," and "disrespect." The possibility of feeling socially invoked pain as an intrinsic product of our nervous system also reinforces the idea that human sociality is a necessary sociality and suggests that our species potentials and constraints—physiological, cognitive, and emotion-al—were selected for in environments where group cooperation was vital.[4] It follows that humans are likely to possess potentials, that is, capacities that can be expected to develop in most environments, for assessing social resources and social threats to which our stress system may then respond (e.g., Flinn et al. 2005).

It is a mixed historical blessing that humans appear able to restrict their sense of just who those others worth paying attention to will be, at least at some times and in some places (e.g., Boyd and Richerson 2008:316–18). This has not been such a time or place for the Aboriginal people of Numbulwar. As Austin-Broos and M. Tonkinson have observed elsewhere on the continent, whitefellas have demanded the attention of Aboriginal people through the exercise of their disproportionate power and their possession of vast and seemingly wonderful material resources. Too often, however, Aboriginal attention encounters forms of social exclusion, in particular, a perceived unwillingness on the part of whitefellas to share. In attending to the larger sociality, Aboriginal people have become, both to others and to themselves, just that, "Aboriginal." Their "primordial identity" has been complicated by an "ethnicity" that occupies a subordinated and, often, denigrated place in the social hierarchy. Their cultural self has been interpenetrated by an "Aboriginal identity" accompanied by feelings that do them no good, socially invoked pain that contributes to their premature morbidity and mortality.

That many non-Indigenous people care whether or not Aboriginal people fall ill and die far earlier than they might is, as I see it, one of the strengths of the Western way of being. Greater Australia, however, for all its good intentions, has nevertheless engaged in decades, if not centuries, of interventions into Aboriginal lives that too often have been ill advised, inadequately funded, and ineffective. The direction I would take for making the world a better place for both indigenous and non-indigenous people would be to ask just what "sharing" means and how genuine sharing might be achieved. I am not advocating a return to "primitive communism." Nor do I think that sharing is limited to the equitable distribution of resources; I sense that it must also include some kind of mutual acknowledgment and dedication to a shared future. Whatever sharing might be, understanding how we might engage the depth of its possibility seems necessary to our times.

Notes

Chapter 1

1. Community-specific summaries of morbidity and mortality for remote communities such as Numbulwar do not exist. Taylor et al. (2000) have gone to considerable pains to create a profile of morbidity and mortality at Ngurkurr, a community located 155 kilometers to the southwest of Numbulwar with which the people of Numbulwar have long had historical and social ties. According to their estimate, and these authors are careful to emphasize the conditional quality of their data, "there are 4.5 times more deaths in Ngurkurr than would be expected if the mortality profile observed for the total Australian population applied." This figure is "slightly higher" than the death rate of "Indigenous people in the Northern Territory as a whole" (80).

   For Numbulwar, I must rely on more impressionistic material for an overview of the health status of people in this community. Nothing I have seen leads me to believe this diverges from what is indicated by continent-wide statistics. An example of this is provided by even superficial knowledge of the health status and related circumstances of the twenty Aboriginal people that I interviewed for this project. Two years after the fieldwork, three were dead while two others had recovered, at least partially, from serious illness, one from tuberculosis and another from kidney disease. During the study period, one interviewee's husband died, as did the adult son of another. None of the ill or dying had reached the age of sixty-five and most were many years younger. Thus nearly a third of this sample, at a minimum, had been touched by the kinds of events that generate the statistics of disproportionate Indigenous illness and death. If the people I interviewed depart in any way from the characteristics of the town's population in general, this would be due to their greater literacy, ability to speak Aboriginal English or the more conventional Australian English, and involvement in religious activities (whether those of the Anglican Church or the Indigenous religion).

2. I refer in particular to versions of schema theory that have been developed along with the use of connectionist modeling in cognitive psychology and advances in neuroscience on the workings of brain synapses. Examples of the use of these models by psychological/cognitive anthropologists may be found in Strauss and Quinn (1994; 1997) and D'Andrade (1995).

3. I include the following as examples of this literature: Bateson 1972; Hinton 1999; Lakoff and Johnson 1980, 1999; Linger 2005; Scheper-Hughes and Lock 1987; Shore 1988; Super and Harkness 1986. There are, of course, many others.
4. These risk factors included high cholesterol and blood pressure, smoking and "others," i.e., "height, body mass, exercise, glucose tolerance" (Wilkinson 1996:65).
5. I use the terms "whitefellas" and "blackfellas" in this work, reflecting the "folk categories of race" (Cowlishaw 2004:10) used at Numbulwar.
6. To do so entirely is an impossible task. The manner in which an anthropologist might do so to a productive degree has been the source of a substantial literature. Readers will find discussions of the issue in one guise or another in many, if not all, of the ethnographies they pick up, especially, perhaps, those that have been published since 1980. And, of course, anthropologists vary in their capacity to identify and suspend their own ideas.
7. All the names used for people at Numbulwar are pseudonyms except those from published historical material used in chapter three.
8. This comment no doubt raises the question of just how one reports back to "a community" of at least 800 people. I presented a talk on preliminary findings to the Numbulwar Council and gave it copies of a CD containing all the photos I had taken of people at Numbulwar since 1977. (Many of these had been lodged previously with the Australian Institute of Aboriginal and Torres Strait Islander Studies' photo collection.) I presented these preliminary findings informally to Aboriginal people not on the Council who had consistently provided me with material over the study period, inserting them in our conversations. I offered to give presentations at the School and the Clinic, in appreciation of the considerable help I had received from people in both institutions, but neither offer was accepted as teachers and health personnel were pressed for time during my visit, in part because the team for the "Board of Inquiry into the Protection of Aboriginal Children from Sexual Abuse" (the bureaucratic step that preceded "the intervention") was visiting that week. During this trip, I was able to ask people for permission to use texts that were not acquired in interviews and to publish photographs I had taken during the research period.
9. I recorded interviews with paper and pencil as people spoke using a form of shorthand I have devised over the years for this purpose. As soon as possible afterward, I reconstructed these notes, which were sometimes almost word for word replications of what people said, but not, of course, always. These reconstructions are what are presented in this book. In a few cases I have deleted repetitions and brief departures from the subject at hand. I have also altered some details that might reveal the identity of speakers, e.g., their kin relationship with me. In making these alterations I have tried, insofar as possible, to minimize distortion, e.g., a blue vehicle might become a black one, a sister might become an aunt.

Texts from interviews are indicated as: (Lily 2003). Comments and conversations recorded some time after the fact in my journals are indicated as: (2004:VI:48). Though I attempted to remember exact words and phrases when I had a chance to make these notes, I was not, of course, always able to do so. These even more than the interview texts should be regarded as "best" approximations.

10. I am reminded here of Frake's (1994) comment that:

> Ethnography...is a very hard thing to do. It can be methodologically messy, socially embarrassing, psychologically upsetting, ethically uncertain, and physically dangerous. But it can also be tremendously revealing of the complex entanglements that enmesh the mind with the cultural, social, and physical worlds within which it works.

I feel particularly aware of the ethical uncertainty just mentioned, when it is time to use the texts I have so painstakingly collected. In this study, the information sheet I presented (verbally) to all interviewees included the following statement: "If you are worrying somebody could guess you told me something and you don't want me to write something you said, tell me and I will not put it in any paper."

One interviewee asked me not to use an account she gave me. With the promised use of pseudonyms and attempts to disguise the identity of both tellers and subjects of statements and stories, I feel comfortable using material from interview-derived texts. But what of statements overheard or winnowed from conversations I had when I was not explicitly acting as an anthropologist, i.e., with pad of paper and pencil in hand, though my identity as such is common knowledge? Here I find things can, at times, be ethically murky. Significant information may be personal or contained within an account that felt intimate in the telling. This is where I often feel torn between ethical concerns and the need to present pertinent and compelling material. On my trip in 2007, I was able to ask four women who had worked with me in the course of the study if it would be alright for me to write about several such incidents that I had witnessed or about accounts they had given me, with the usual promises of anonymity and confidentiality. Three of the four women said I could use the events/accounts. One demurred and the interaction I had witnessed, though pertinent, is one I do not use. It is easier to decide to use material when similar information is heard, or overheard, from several people and presenting it can be done in general terms; e.g. "Several people said that All Star had come to Numbulwar selling 999 channels" or "Some of the accounts of this murder focused on sorcery, that is, what is today being called 'black magic' by people at Numbulwar." I might also note that use of conversational texts from all three sources is standard practice in ethnography.

11. Identifying details in this text have been changed. It is being used with the, now adult, speaker's knowledge and permission. I might note here that in 2007 when we had this conversation, the speaker continued to

attribute her vomiting to "walking in the hot sun," not to the content of what she related, though I invited her to do so. This may or may not indicate a failure of my empathic effort (see Hollan 2008; Kirmayer 2008).

12 Though expressed in the language of an earlier anthropology of emotions, the following remark by Huntington and Metcalf (1979) seems pertinent:

> Emotions may be vague and irrational, but when the analyst knows the culture and the particular participants, and has him- or herself shared in the events, and furthermore, is extremely scrupulous of the level of verifiability of each piece of evidence, then the study of the emotional aspects of life yields great dividends. (34–5)

Chapter 2

1. Readers who wish to look up Numbulwar on the Internet may do so by simply searching for "Numbulwar."

2. The concept of "culture change" and associated ideas of "intercultural" encounters and situations have long been a part of anthropological thinking, though the emphasis they receive has varied over the decades. For example, years ago, in their discussion of the "study of values in five cultures," Vogt and Albert (1966a) mention "a de facto intercultural system, with important dynamics of its own" (25). These dynamics are discussed in a chapter titled "Intercultural relations" in the "study of values" collection (Vogt and Albert 1966b). I also refer readers to Hinkson's (2005) discussion of Stanner's "intercultural" field experiences in the north of Australia and to Reay's (1949) ethnography of rural people in north-western New South Wales.

3. Katherine is a Northern Territory town of some 9,000 people, about 370 kilometers, almost due west, from Numbulwar.

4. Though Merlan (2005) draws in particular on Sahlins, Bourdieu, and Voloshinov to "deal with question of difference, boundedness, reproduction and transformation" (172), I find her treatment of the intercultural, particularly the ways she emphasizes the relational and processual qualities of subjectivity and links these to cultural reproduction and change, reminiscent of Spiro's (1951) thinking on the relationship between culture and personality. Arguing for their near identity—"the development of personality and the acquisition of culture are one and the same process" (31)—one of his conclusions is that "the culture of any society is not the sum of the individual cultural heredities, nor is it the direct manifestation of the total cultural heritage; it is, rather, the product of the interaction of all the individuals in the society" (41). And then, because of the inevitable difference in individual experience, "Culture, therefore, is constantly changing, as new behavioural patterns arise through interaction and older ones fall into disuse. Culture, then is

heterogeneous and changing, for culture is the product of interacting individuals and not the reflection of a determinate cultural heritage" (42).

5. The label "Nunggubuyu" is used to refer to an Indigenous language,
that of the ancestors of Numbulwar's majority population. It is translated, however, as "people who speak Wubuy" (Heath 1982:126).

6. The English spoken by many at Numbulwar is referred to as "Aboriginal
English." Eades (1993) has suggested that Aboriginal English should be
understood as a dialect of English that varies from other versions of it in
systematic ways. These ways in turn may vary across the Australian continent because the different Indigenous languages affecting the gram-
matical structure of Aboriginal English may themselves vary. As Walsh
(1993) has observed, the differences between Australian and Aboriginal
English may be subtle ones. Eades (1993), e.g., has observed that the
meanings of "shame" in Aboriginal English "has no simple equivalent"
in Australian English (188).

7. CDEP is referred to as CDP by both whitefellas and blackfellas at
Numbulwar. According to Sanders (2005), the CDEP scheme, initiated
in the late 1970s and administered by the Department of Aboriginal
Affairs, was implemented in remote communities nationwide by the early
1990s; it was a program that did not replace unemployment benefits, but
provided money in addition to them. Designed for Indigenous people in
remote communities, CDEP provided salaries for workers doing up to
twenty hours of work a week. Activities considered to be valuable by the
community were those usually funded.

8. At the time of my fieldwork in 1977 and 1978, various people at
Numbulwar identified themselves, or were identified by other Aboriginal
people, as Numburindi, Nunggubuyu, Ingura, Wandarang, Mara,
Ngandi, or Ridharngu. Numburindi refers to a group of people associ-
ated with the land north of Numbulwar in the general area of Wurindi.
The language once spoken by these people is Wubuy. The labels Ngandi,
Wandarang, and Mara identify languages once or still spoken by groups
inhabiting stretches of land south of Numburindi countries, and to the
south of Numbulwar. Numbulwar itself is located in what was once a
Wandarang speaking area.

By 1977, and probably much earlier, groups that once spoke
Ridharngu, Mara, Wandarang, and Dha'i (and possibly Dhangu) had
adopted Wubuy as their first language. These groups referred to themselves as Nunggubuyu. Thus, people from what was once a Wandarang
speaking area might refer to themselves as Wandarang on one occasion
and as Nunggubuyu on another.

Keen (1995, 2000) has argued that the term "clan" is an inadequate
and distorting translation of Yolngu *ba:purru*. I use the term for similar
sorts of social divisions at Numbulwar primarily because the Aboriginal
people of Numbulwar speak of their "clan." People are said to be of a
certain clan because they come from a country associated with that clan.
Usually, this is their father's country (Burbank 1980:24).

The population of Numbulwar who derive from Wubuy speakers may be divided into eleven clans, three of which are said to be non-Numburindi: the Numamudidi, once Wandarang speakers; the Wurramarra, originally Anindiljuagwa (Ingura) speakers from Bickerton Island; and the Mangurra, once Ridharngu speakers whose territory lies just north of Harris Creek, near the Walker River. Three other clans, the Nunggayiynbalayn, Magurri, and Nungguldulbuy, are identified as Numburindi on the ground that their countries are in the general area of Wurindi, although it was also said that they were once Wandarang, Mara, or Dha'i speakers. The remaining patriclans, Nglami, Nunggumajbar/Nunggulngulgu, Murrungun, Nundhirribala, and Nunggargalung, are identified as "proper real Nunggubuyu mob" (Burbank 1980:1–3).

9. I was told by a whitefella of long acquaintance with Numbulwar that its mail was sent to Katherine, then sent, or returned, to Darwin for delivery to the town. Once it was actually flown from Katherine, hence the address of "CMB 17, via Katherine," but as the airline with this route was no longer in business at the time of the study, the mail was flown out of Darwin with airlines that flew to Groote Eylandt. From there it was brought in by MAF (Mission Aviation Fellowship) planes.

   Telephones and fax machines were relatively new to the town. In 1977 it was possible to send a telegram to and from Numbulwar, but there was no guarantee it would be received as I was to discover on more than one occasion. In 1981, the Council office had obtained a radio telephone that did not allow simultaneous talking and listening, requiring the speaker to manipulate a switch between the two modes. During the years of this study, I watched the Telstra helicopter stationed at Groote Eylandt land and take off from the old, deserted basketball court that I could see from my veranda. In 2003, many of the people that I know had phones in their homes. By the next year, most if not all of the phones had been turned off because of nonpayment of bills. In 2007, one of the women I know told me that she had been receiving calls on her mobile from Telstra that made her "nervous." They were asking her to pay the $1,000 or so that she owed from 2003. My impression was that only the whitefella houses still had landlines by 2007; Aboriginal people used mobiles. "Prepaid" arrangements allowed them to use their phones when they had money to buy "credit" and not run up debt when they did not.

10. I have subsequently been informed that by May 2008, management of Numbulwar's shop had been taken over by the ALPA (Arnhem Land Progress Association).

11. There were, however, reports of hunger during the study: "Sometimes people come and visit, but you know they want food" (ITU 2005); "I didn't have any food yesterday, but *nga marig* [my daughter] gave me $50 for sugar, flour, tea leaf, baking powder" (2005 III:15).

Children, I was told by householders on occasion, hadn't gone to school because they didn't "eat any breakfast." Often my visitors, primarily women, children, and female adolescents, said they were "hungry." I am not sure, however, if a statement such as, "I am hungry, auntie" is a report of hunger so much as it is a form of "demand sharing" (discussed at length in chapter four), action that may be motivated as much by the desire to establish and/or maintain a relationship as it is to satisfy a physical need.

12. The Church Missionary Society maintained a no alcohol rule during their years of control of the Rose River Mission. I was told by a long-term resident missionary on my first field trip that the rule had only rarely been violated. On that trip, however, I knew of thirteen occasions when alcohol had been brought to Numbulwar (Burbank 1980). This situation seemed to have been reversed by the time of my 1981 visit. Numbulwar had been declared "dry" following a Northern Territory Liquor Commission consultation with the community. I assumed at the time that the new signs I had seen at nearby airstrips and on the road into Numbulwar were having the desired effect. They proclaimed that any vehicle (including planes) found transporting alcohol would be impounded (see Burbank 1994:62–3).

13. GEMCO, according to its website in 2008, is jointly owned by BHP Billiton and Anglo American Corporation.

14. Six of the respondents included the words "homesick" or "boring" in their replies. While I understand their meaning of "homesick" to be similar to mine, in Aboriginal usage "boring" often seems to contain an emphasis on sociality not generally found in its Western meaning (see also Musharbash 2007). For example,

Boring when you see community real hot and steaming. People say, 'I'm too hot, it's boring, nobody walking around, it's too dead'. I can't walk around. I stay home, listen to tape or DVD or culture tape. If they don't see people walking around, they call it "boring." They want to see people everywhere so it's gonna look nice. (Emma 2005)

Of course, there are many people walking around in "the city," but clearly not just any people will do, as Simone's (2004) comment makes clear: "Feel like homesick, thinking about my family." There was also a perception on the part of some of these women that life in the city was dangerous.

Something might happen [in the city]. Car accident or someone gonna stab me with the knife. It's dangerous. If you go and see the Long Grass People, they give you shit for money and they stab you with the knife. They got the knife in the pocket. You gotta be careful to yourself. (Kinsey 2005)

"Long Grass People" are Aboriginal people who travel to Darwin and camp on its outskirts or in relatively un-built areas, such as wastelands or parks; they are associated at Numbulwar with the activities of drinking and drug taking. In 2005, one of the funerals I attended was held for a man who had long lived in Darwin. He had died after being stabbed by another Aboriginal man. Kinsey, it appears, was thinking of this incident in her reply.

15. While the population of Numbulwar may be said to have numbered 800 more or less regular residents during the years of this study, another 200 or so people might be visiting at any given time. These, as often as not, were people from nearby places such as Ngukurr, Borroloola, Bickerton Island, or Groote Eylandt, places where unmarried people at Numbulwar might find a spouse, as might have at least one of their parents, if their parents had not themselves come from one of these locales. And so, as visitors from Ngukurr and Groote and Bickerton come to Numbulwar, people who normally reside at Numbulwar go to Bickerton or Groote or Ngukurr. Some of these visits, both to and from Numbulwar, may be more permanent than others. Shapiro (1979) has mentioned the willingness with which women of northeast Arnhem Land move to live with their married daughters (24). Undoubtedly, some of Numbulwar's visitors and travelers were people who had come or gone to be with children, parents, grandparents, and other kin.

Weekly scheduled and charter flights by MAF and motorized dinghies enabled frequent short- as well as long-term visits between Groote and Bickerton islands and Numbulwar. The road running between Numbulwar and Ngukurr had been improved over the years and the time it takes to travel between the two communities has decreased. Having spent between four and six hours on this road on previous fieldtrips, I found myself disbelieving the report that it could be traversed in a mere half hour, but I did not have occasion to find out if this were true. Recently, travelers have mentioned a two-hour journey. Even during the wet season, when once the road might have been impassible for months, people seem able to travel between Ngukurr and Numbulwar, though I was told of at least one occasion in 2007 when the water in the creeks it crossed was just too high to do so. Vehicle ownership has also increased from earlier times, facilitating visits between these two communities. Access to vehicles and boats has also enabled people to bring alcohol and cannabis into the community in quantities unknown in the past.

People at Numbulwar also travel, usually by plane or vehicle, to more distant remote communities such as Borroloola, Bulman, and Oenpelli. They also travel to larger towns and cities such as Katherine, Darwin, and Adelaide. Many of these trips are made so that people can attend ceremonies or festivals, such as the Barunga Festival, held in a community about eighty kilometers southeast of Katherine. Occasions for trips might be commercial: to sell art or buy supplies for painting and basketwork. People might also travel to Darwin or Katherine in order to buy a vehicle. Occasions for trips might be work or family related: escorting children to a school event in Katherine or an ill person to a medical facility in Darwin or Adelaide. People might also travel in order to attend various religious or political events. Circumcisions and other ceremonies drew people from Numbulwar to various other parts of the Northern Territory. Nungalinya College in Darwin holds classes for religious study and Bible translation workshops that some people regularly attend. In 2004, the Council president went to Brisbane to participate in an Indigenous leadership workshop. Training for people who worked in the school, clinic, or Council office sometimes took them to Batchelor College, located outside of Darwin. Rarely, such training took them even further afield. Four women from Numbulwar attended courses at Curtin University in Perth, Western Australia, during the study period. The Yilila Band made more than one trip to Darwin during this time and in 2007 visited Ireland to perform. Numbulwar's Red Flag Dancers have performed at the Garma festival in the Yirrkala/Nhulunbuy area, in Darwin for the Telstra Awards, and in Sydney for the 2000 Olympics.

16. As a part of the intervention, a portion of welfare payments have been "quarantined" to ensure that these funds will not be spent on alcohol and drugs and other items judged to be nonessential, a judgment that may not be shared by Aboriginal people .

17. I was not present for funerals where the deceased was extremely young and the death unexpected, though funerals occasioned by such deaths did occur during the study period. The six funerals that I did attended were held for two women and four men. I attended two during a three-month field trip in 2003 and one during a similar length stay in 2004. That year, I missed at least three that occurred at the beginning of the year, and one that was held a day after I left the town. In 2005, I attended three. I heard of others that occurred during the study years, and during the time of writing, from phone calls to me when I was back in Perth. In addition to funerals held at Numbulwar, people who reside there often traveled to nearby communities in order to attend funerals of kin.

18. For a discussion of death, funerals, and sorcery in the nearby community of Ngukurr, see O'Donnell (2007), especially pages 270–85. For a discussion of sorcery at Ngukurr, see Senior (2003), especially pages 164–75.

19. Much of the ritual paraphernalia associated with clans is sacred and secret. Songs of this kind would not be performed for an audience of children, women, and uninitiated men.

20. I do not know how much people hear of these sermons. Both inside and outside the church speakers must compete with the sounds of conversation, babies' cries, and occasional dog fights.

21. Music is often played at a very high volume. This may be due, at least in part, to the hearing impairment occasioned by ear infection. Hearing problems are reported to be widespread in remote communities such as Numbulwar (ABS 2005).

22. I have identified, along with my coauthors, a similar emphasis on the importance of family in mortuary practices in Indigenous communities across Australia (see Burbank et al. 2008). This, of course, continues the emphasis on "relatedness" (Myers 1986) in Aboriginal sociality.

23. For example, in 1988, Numbulwar was visited by a Christian group from Groote Eylandt who brought with them the practice of "action," singing accompanied by a dance routine to popular music with Christian themes, such as those sung by Emmylou Harris. This visit coincided with an outbreak of petrol sniffing that had seemed to entice many, if not the majority of adolescents in the community. In the days following this visit, most if not all of the adolescents were engaged in "action" for hours every day, to judge by the music I could hear, and the epidemic of petrol sniffing came to an end.

24. Majiwi here refers to two Aboriginal communities on Groote Eylandt. One of these, Angurugu, another former CMS mission, is called "Groote" by people at Numbulwar. Her opinion that these communities were "forgetting" their culture was shared by other people I know and, indeed, men from Numbulwar often traveled to Groote Eylandt to sing at funerals there.

25. Strauss and Quinn (1997) see "social evaluation" as a part of enculturation and as the source of emotionally weighted lessons (94–5). That is, learning that some aspects of experience are either valued or devalued by significant others may evoke strong emotions. Hence, feelings of anxiety and security, or eventually their culturally specific emotional manifestations, become a part of schemas that ground our sense of the "natural" and the "moral" and motivate our behavior.

26. No one, a woman herself included, should bring her sexual, reproductive, or eliminatory functions to the attention of any of her adult brothers as identified by the classificatory kinship system. In the past, the public location of toilet blocks, the only toilet facilities available for most Aboriginal people until the 1980s, made conformity with this etiquette quite challenging at times. Women, however, developed strategies to deal with their new circumstances, for example, grabbing a towel and saying they were going to take a shower. Nevertheless, women also spoke of the discomfort of full bladders that could not be emptied because a brother was present (see Burbank 1985). During this study, Majiwi (2004) mentioned that *mirriri* was now considered "domestic violence": "They [brothers] been slowed down by the police. It's like domestic violence, we call the police. Police can come here straight away now. That's why they don't bother to chase us, just walk away if [they] hear a rude word."

27. The genealogical idea of "close" was explained to me with reference to a shared ancestor. For example, two people might be close because they were "one granny" (Burbank 1980). R. Tonkinson's (1978) remarks on Aboriginal kinship provide an easy means of grasping the mode of classification at Numbulwar. Two principles are central. First "same sex" siblings are treated as equivalent, for example, one's mother's sister would also be called "mother." Second, "the classifying principle can be applied to a theoretically infinite range; the web of kinship thus extends far beyond consanguineal and local group limits to include the most distant of kin and former strangers" (43). Thus, once I was adopted by my "sister," that is, made her equivalent, anyone at Numbulwar could easily calculate his or her relationship to me.

28. Musharbash's (2008) treatment of sleeping arrangements at Yuendumu suggested this equation to me. By recording hundreds of sleeping arrangements over years of participant observation, she found that they could be read as representations of the ways in which people felt about each other. In a household, e.g., people who had been arguing would sleep further apart from each other than they did when they were on better terms. More generally, in conjunction with Grady (1997), Lakoff and Johnson (1999) identify "intimacy is closeness" as a primary metaphor, i.e., a mental structure arising from early interactions with the world that enables understanding of more complex experience:

    Intimacy Is Closeness
      Subjective Experience: Intimacy
      Sensorymotor Experience: Being physically close
      Example: "We've been *close* for years but we're beginning to *drift apart*."
      Primary Experience: Being physically close to people you are intimate with. (50)

29. Although *balanda* is a word that originates with Yolngu speakers in north east Arnhem Land, it was sometimes used at Numbulwar by both whitefellas, as in this quote, and blackfellas.

Chapter 3

1. The materials for this chapter are scant in two respects. First, very little is known about Aboriginal health prior to European colonization. Reconstructions must rely on the impressionistic reports of early contacts (largely from the southern part of the continent), knowledge of hunter-gatherer health more generally, and skeletal remains. Scholars using these, very tentatively, conclude that Aboriginal people surviving the first five years of life were generally healthy and well nourished. They suffered little from infectious and chronic disease. They were more likely to suffer injury or death from accidents and, occasionally,

violence (Beck 1985:6–11; Franklin and White 1991:3; Saggers and Gray 1991:36–42). Historical records are also scarce. I have made use of the few I have been able to locate. Professor John Bern (personal communication) and Dr. Rosemary O'Donnell (2007:9–10), both of whom work at Ngukurr, have also noted the dearth of historical materials for this area.

2. The Macassans might also have brought smallpox to the Nunggubuyu, according to Campbell (1997). On the basis of her review of historical and medical records, she is convinced that "Asian visitors, probablyMacassans" infected Aboriginal people with this disease (294). Of the epidemics that followed, she suggests that: "The failure of traditional medicine, bereavement and melancholy, the fear of impending disaster and fears about unfulfilled obligations to their dead all suggest a devastating loss of morale in affected groups" (295).

    I have, however, no evidence of smallpox arriving with the Macassans who met the Nunggubuyu. The Nunggubuyu texts on Macassans collected by Heath (1980) make no mention of illness but rather focus largely on positive events, such as learning how to make dugout canoes (530–50). One text concerns the actions of what Heath refers to as "Macassan culture heroes." He notes that "Macassans are the specialty of the Nun-dhiribala clan (Yirija moiety) in particular, from whom 'sail' (dhumbala) is the major wungubal song cycle" (550). The principal dance performed by the Red Flag Dancers during the study years was *dhumbala* (a word of Macassan origin according to Heath).

3. We must also consider the possibility that prior to colonization, individuals may have suffered considerable stress. Warner (1937), for example, writing of Yolngu people during a time that includes accounts of a recent pre-mission period, discusses abduction and murder (58, 66, 71). Women, including pregnant ones, might be abducted and their abduction might be accompanied by the murder of their husbands. It is hard to imagine circumstances in which such experiences would not be stressful. Similarly, I might posit co-wife hostility, a well-documented phenomenon in Aboriginal Australia (e.g., Burbank 1994), as a source of considerable and continuing stress. Drawing primarily on Warner's ethnography, (1937), I have suggested that a few men in Aboriginal groups of the past might have been highly aggressive individuals, as is likely to be the case in any community, at any time. Wives and children of these men may have found life more stressful than wives and children of those with more mild-mannered temperaments (Burbank 2000). With the advent of colonization, however, according to my argument, it would be the exceptional individual who did not experience considerable and continuing stress.

4. Note that when the mission was built it was located several kilometers from this sacred area and not in this man's country (Cole 1982:28).

5. This is only the first part of Madi's account of the mission's establishment and I have not included the word for word translations of Heath's (1980) texts.

6. A recent study by Brown et al. (2008) asks a similar question about Cherokee and White youth in Appalachia (United States). In their ethnographic approach to use of the SSS, a measure of "subjective social status," they are interested in the "underspecified determinants" (290) of subjective judgment as opposed to the standard components of this and similar measures, e.g., occupation, education, and income. They assume, in essence, that we cannot know beforehand just what criteria people will use when they compare themselves to others.

7. This interpretation of the experience of housing differentials should in no way be regarded as incompatible with accounts such as Bailie's (2007) where more immediate connections between housing adequacy and health are posited. For example, he points out that nutrition can be adversely affected if houses do not provide adequate and hygienic means for storing and preparing food (212).

8. The analysis excluded all spontaneous abortions, stillbirths, neonatal and infant deaths, and births where the father was known to be different from the father of the preceding child.

9. In her cross-cultural study of "conjugal dissolution," Betzig (1989) found infertility second only to adultery in frequency as a reason for divorce (662).

10. Observing that it is difficult to ascertain if pre-colonized Australian populations were relatively small "due to low birthrates or high infant mortality," Saggers and Gray (1991) evaluate the probable validity of Cowlishaw's argument, finding several factors in its support (23). These include Abbie's (1976) comparison of hemoglobin levels in remote dwelling Aboriginal people and "European" Australians. Only in the latter group was a sex difference found, i.e., European women had lower hemoglobin levels than did European men. The absence of a sex difference in the Aboriginal group may be interpreted to mean that these women had "less frequent and shorter menstrual periods," indicating "less frequent ovulation" and hence lower fertility (24). Saggers and Gray also mention dietary restrictions to which Aboriginal women were subjected, patterns of breast-feeding that may have reduced ovulation, and the possibility that genital operations such as subincision reduced male fertility. I am not aware of this operation ever having been a part of the series of male inductions into the religious life of the Nunggubuyu.

   In the literature addressing hunter gatherer fertility in general, Bentley et al. (1993) have pointed out that: "[F]orager, horticultural, and agricultural groups are all characterized by a high degree of heterogeneity in their fertility rates, and that it is not possible to predict fertility rates on the basis of subsistence technology alone" (276–7).

   Nevertheless, following an analysis of natural-fertility populations, they concluded that "the intensification of subsistence technology is associated with increases in fertility...Higher fertility is primarily associated with the intensification of agriculture." While the people of Numbulwar have not become agriculturalists, their way of life upon settlement at Rose River Mission increasingly became supported by the intensified technology associated with industrial societies.

With respect to fertility, Bentley et al. (2001) have emphasized women's subsistence activities as "crucial given the relationship between women's energetic output and gonadal function." Factors to consider here would include the distance women travel, the loads they are required to carry (including dependent children), and the energy required by daily subsistence tasks, e.g., digging for roots. An additional factor is "the level of temperatures to be endured" (Bentley 1985:86). This factor may well have affected the energetics of foraging in a climate that is hot and humid during most of the year. Though this literature makes it clear this is not always the case in a shift from a foraging to a horticultural subsistence strategy, the energetic demands of settled life for Numbulwar's women would seem to have been reduced considerably. Heat and humidity have much less of an effect on someone being driven less than half a kilometer to the shop than on someone gathering food in areas that may be some kilometers from camp.

Chapter 4

1. A slender body does not seem to invite the approval and admiration it receives in segments of Western society. I have been, on occasion, referred to as a "bone fella," clearly not a compliment. On the other hand, people have remarked favorably when I have been seen to be getting "fat." Later in this chapter the reader will note Carmel's comment in the discussion of ganja and grog, associating cannabis use with weight loss. This is, perhaps, as much a sign of disapproval of the practice as an observation that people at Numbulwar who smoke a lot of ganja lose weight. Some of the people identified to me as dedicated ganja smokers were indeed thinner than many other Numbulwar residents. It could reflect their use of money to buy ganja instead of food.

2. I first heard of the suicide in this account in 1997. While people at Numbulwar have subsequently lost kin to suicide, these deaths took place in other communities. In 2008, another suicide occurring at Numbulwar was reported to me, though not confirmed. There have also been numerous suicide attempts at Numbulwar since the loss Carmel mentions. These cases have been described as impulsive, attention-seeking acts that could have resulted, by accident, in death, but fortunately have not. Carmel (2003) describes one such attempt: "[A man] tried to hang himself from a power pole by my place. He was drunk, off his head. I just pulled him down, and said, 'You do it somewhere else. I don't want my grandkids to copy you.'"

3. Hand signs distinguish smoking tobacco from smoking ganja. For tobacco, the first two fingers are held together slightly above the mouth. For ganja, the thumb and first finger are pinched together slightly

below the mouth. The thumb near the mouth with first finger pointing forward, parallel, more or less, to the face is the sign for *boddle*, what is known in some Western circles as a "bong," an instrument made from a plastic soda bottle for smoking cannabis.

4. "Touristing" means going to town drinking and smoking ganja.
5. "Trouble" is a word used to indicate aggression, including sorcery. Other forms of misbehavior, such as running off with an unacceptable marriage partner, are often introduced in a conversation with the words "[name] making trouble." These are acts that are expected to provoke aggression whether verbal, physical, or supernatural (Burbank 1994:51). Sometimes the word "problem" appeared to be used as a synonym for both trouble and "make trouble" in the Aboriginal English I heard during the study period. At other times it seemed to be used to signify a state of affairs of which trouble might or might not be a part.
6. Another woman might also have been thinking along the same lines:

    AW: Young people here doing it [black magic]
    VKB: What for?
    AW: Money, they pay them. Maybe somebody forcing them to do it. (2003:XII:58)
7. This analytic move is inspired by Hutchins' (1987) treatment of the Trobriand myth of Baroweni as an instantiation of a psychodynamically repressed schema, *I negligently killed my dead parent* (284). In proposing that *other people can make us dead* is an analogue of *other people can make us feel bad,* I believe I have satisfied the criterion he has set for such a relationship and in doing so have at least postulated if not identified the underlying schema and its source:

    > Support for the analogical interpretation requires a single schema that, when instantiated in different ways, generates the proposition of the myth as well as the proposition describing the conditions of life. Such a schema would be a structure composed of more general terms than those found in the instances to be accounted for. To discover the underlying schema, we examine the terms in the proposition of the myth and the description of the relevant bits of life and find for them the most specific category that is general enough to contain the set of terms. (280)
8. In contrast, McKnight (2005) says, in reference to Aboriginal people on Mornington Island, that sorcery explanations of death have been supplanted by explanations that refer to excess drinking, "In the past the elders asserted that people 'did not die for nothing' and nowadays that still holds, but instead of dying from sorcery people die from alcohol" (211). His observation raises the question of why sorcery continued to have such apparent psychological resilience at Numbulwar. Even people who initially seemed to accept a doctor's or coroner's explanation for a death would later talk of sorcery as the cause, often with considerable feeling. A first guess about this resilience would be that "black magic" provides a more adequate explanation; it accounts for more cases than

ascriptions of excessive drinking can, given the patterns of morbidity and mortality in this community.

9. Nor would such feelings be experienced identically by different people, or by people in different communities. See Reddy (1997; 2001) for a discussion of the ways in which what he calls emotion discourses interact with our species' capacities to feel.

10. Sutton (2009) might see the teenage girl's action as "cruelling," the infliction of pain on infants and small children with acts such as slapping, pinching, or biting. These acts, usually performed by kin, appear "to be done ostensibly for the purpose of encouraging self-assertion, although deeper and less functional explanations to do with repressed anger and jealousy on the part of the instigator are probably relevant" (111). While the motive may be as he suspects, I would maintain that as cruelling is often followed by acts that seem to console a child, the infliction of pain only serves to increase the child's emotional connection to family, that is, the comfort, and its source become as memorable as the experience of pain (see Quinn 2005c).

11. Fiske's (1992) ideas about the "cognitive structure of social relationships" (713) are relevant here. Assuming "that people are fundamentally sociable" (689), Fisk has abstracted four models from numerous experimental and ethnographic examples "that generate most kinds of social interaction, evaluation, and affect" (689). Among these is one that he calls "equality matching," a model that enables comparison via "the use of operations of addition and subtraction to assess imbalance" (690). While he "gives culture a crucial role" in the expression of these models, he sees them as universally present in human sociality, "endogenous products of the human mind" (690). Here I might note the comment that:

> Many findings in behavioural, developmental, neuropsychological and neuroimaging studies converge to suggest a variety of representation of numbers and a variety of processes engaged in numerical inference... [that enable]... the capacity to judge relative amounts. (Boyer and Barrett 2005:111)

I might also note the numerous observations that people are "highly averse" to receiving less that others (e.g., Fiske 1992:704) and related lines of thought pursued in the literature on "strong reciprocity" (e.g., Fehr and Henrich 2003) and "inequity aversion" (e.g., Bräuer et al. 2006).

12. The "baby bonus" came from the Australian Federal Government, which gave $3,000 to women upon the birth of a child.

Chapter 5

1. Driessen (1999) has observed that "there is now a burgeoning literature on 'identity,' to the point that any scholar...writing about this

broad theme runs the risk of overlooking relevant literature" (432). Discussions of "self" in anthropological usage are also in plentiful supply. The relatively recent debates that have surrounded self as an anthropological concept (e.g., Shweder and Bourne 1984; Spiro 1993; Wierzbicka 1993) provide useful entrees to this literature.

2. Sökefeld (1999) nominates self as a human universal. He builds his case via a discussion of self as the locus of agency and action. "Action," he says, "requires a self that reflexively monitors the conditions, course, and outcome of action. This reflexivity includes the consciousness of the basic difference between the self and everything else" (430).

Support for the idea of a species-wide potential to develop a sense of self might also be grounded in the idea that not just humans but any animal needs something of the sort we label "self" simply for survival (which, of course, requires action). Panksepp's (1998) discussion of the *periaqueductal gray* (also known as the PAG) of the basic mammalian level of the brain seems relevant here:

> The superior colliculus is especially interesting because it is here that we begin to get a glimmer of the first evolutionary appearance of a sophisticated representation of self. This might be expected simply from the fact that this part of the brain contains multimodal sensory systems designed to elaborate simple orientation responses. In other words, these systems may provide a sense of presence for the animal within its world. (77)

The capacity to perceive "the basic difference between myself and everything else" (Sökefeld 1999:424) would seem to be critical. How could an animal survive without knowing where *it* was?

3. Ever since I have been visiting Numbulwar, the Aboriginal people there have used the contrasting terms whitefellas/blackfella and *wuruwuruj/munanga* or (less often) *dhurdaba*. Heath (1982) translates the singular of the first term in the latter contrast as "human (not animal), Aboriginal (not European)," the second as "white person, European," with *dhurdaba* given as a synonym (252,114). The words "Aborigine" and "Aboriginal person" are used as synonyms of "blackfella" or *wuruwuruj*, the plural of *wuruj*. When Lily and I discussed the questions I might use for the study, she said that "Indigenous person" might be better than "Aboriginal person," when I offered the alternatives, because "that what all the *munanga* [say]" (2003:I:22). I found, however, that most of the people I interviewed tended to use words other than "Indigenous," and so I reverted to "Aboriginal person" or its translations. When people were talking about themselves or others as an "Aboriginal person," they often rubbed their (usually upper) arm, as though to indicate the color of their skin, sometimes also commenting how they had "black" or "brown" skin. Skin color alone, however, is not a sufficient criterion for inclusion in the category *wuruwuruj* (see also Tonkinson 1990).

4. I thank Jim Chisholm for thinking to run Chi-Squares on the positive/negative contrast of interactions and emotions in the Aboriginal and

munanga stories. These revealed that the textual analyses demonstrate significant differences between the stories told about Aboriginal people and *munangas*. Aboriginal/non-Aboriginal identity by statements about positive and negative interactions has a Pearson Chi-Square Value of 6.887 and an Asymp. Significance (two-sided) of .009. Aboriginal/non-Aboriginal Identity by statements about positive and negative emotions has a Pearson Chi-Square Value of 4.335 and an Asymp. Significance (two-sided) of .037.

5. I constructed this question having heard people categorize *munanga* as "good" and "bad" during previous field trips.

6. It may be that Ngalba has had many such experiences and hence this is a fair generalization about whitefellas. On the other hand, her extension of this single experience to whitefella/blackfella relations more generally may be due to an "illusory correlation." According to Hirschfeld (1997): "An illusory correlation is an erroneous inference about the relationship between two classes of events. Specifically, an illusory correlation is the overestimation of the frequency of with which distinctive events co-occur" (66). Infrequent events he says, following Hamilton and Gifford (1976), attract our attention. When two infrequent events co-occur, they attract even greater attention and "people tend to perceive a correlation between them." Negative events occur less often than other kinds of events; minority people, who, by virtue of being in the minority, are encountered by the majority less often as well. Hence the likelihood that a single negative experience with a member of minority will be ascribed to that minority in general.

7. Only the youngest respondent provided a completely positive view of Aboriginal people through *munanga* eyes:

> Maybe they like Aboriginal people. Like maybe they like to invite them to *munanga* place to having supper or talking to them. Maybe *munanga* like the Aborigine people to come with them walking at the beach and maybe the Aboriginal people show them how people going fishing, spearing turtle and dugong. (AW 2005)

It is not clear whether or not this young woman responded as she did in an effort to please me or because this reflected her experience. She had only recently left school, which she had seemed to like—at least during the years I was there for this study. Many of the schoolteachers appeared to have friends among the local people and acted toward their students with kindness and generosity. If this respondent's experience up to the time of the interview had been primarily with teachers such as these, her text might indeed be a reflection of her experience.

8. Merry's negative experience with All Stars might have been exacerbated because it required her to speak English. Alternatively, English may make Merry "nervous" because it is a language she associates with having to speak to All Stars. Here is an excerpt from an interview we did together on another day that year:

VKB: How do you feel when you speak English?
Merry: When I feel like speaking, I speak especially to white people, especially All Stars mob.
VKB: All Stars mob?
Merry: Like asking me for bill and how much I gonna pay. Sometimes I feel nervous when it's hot. I get nervous, little bit, not much. (Merry 2005)

Chapter 6

1. Acciaioli (1981) has observed that "Bourdieu's endeavour seems curiously parallel to that of the Culture and Personality theorists of the 1930s" (31). As Quinn's approach, and mine, spring from that tradition, some readers may now be wondering about parallels between Bourdieu's concept of *habitus* and what I have presented here. Strauss and Quinn (1997:284–5; 1997:44–7) have compared their ideas about cultural cognition with *habitus*. The most obvious and important contrast is that their model of the cultural mind is "neurally inspired," whereas Bourdieu's *habitus* creates a "psychological" space without psychological content. In his scheme of things, it is only internalized culture that receives attention, enabling anthropology to maintain an identity apart from psychology.

2. Convergent evidence of this is provided by the literature on attachment (e.g., Hazan and Shaver 1987) and on transference (e.g., Freud 1989). A compelling argument regarding transference is provided by Westen and Gabbard's (2002a; 2002b) integration of psychoanalytic theories of transference with findings from connectionist modeling.

3. In making this analytic move, I have wondered if I might be falling into the homunculus trap. I am encouraged, however, by Gregg's (1998) efforts. His reworking of Erikson's (1968) ideas about identity in combination with LeVine's (1973) on a genotypic/phenotypic personality distinction provides an example of how a deft analysis of identity and self can avoid this analytic misstep. In Gregg's (1998) scheme, genotypic personality is understood as "an animating core of affective/kinaesthetic tension" and phenotypic personality is seen as a "system of self-representation that interprets these tension and orchestrates their performance" (126). While phenotypic personality might at first glance appear as a centralized controlling agent, Gregg's discussion of "ambiguous symbols in self-representational discourse" makes it clear that this is not the case. These symbols that, in effect, organize the experience of self and others:

   > prove especially suitable for linking affect and cognition. And because subsets of features can evoke different affects...or encode contrasting concepts...they prove suitable for organizing alternative interpretations of inner experiences and social events. (145)

Reading this with schema in mind, we can see symbols being learned in association with experiences of the body in the world, feelings, and other symbols. Depending upon the environmental stimuli to which the person is exposed at the moment, different facets of the learned symbols are attended to and their associated schema are activated creating various, yet constrained, self experiences, all without being orchestrated by a central actor. The emotional and motivational priority that I give to early experience of self with others, while more likely to be activated and hence a part of an experience, can only contribute to it as this schema interacts with other schema that are evoked by the current circumstances.

4. Referring to LeDoux (2002), Quinn (2003) says, "Hormones released during emotional arousal actually strengthen synaptic connections, and emotional arousal organizes and coordinates brain activity, crowding all but the emotionally relevant experience out of consciousness" (148).

5. Even businesses producing services are cast in these terms; e.g., a service is called "our product." We might imagine, in contrast, an educational institution constructed via a "nurturing parent" family metaphor, where the process of "nurturing" is given priority. We might also consider possibilities for businesses organized around a "school" or "family" metaphor, as some probably are.

6. "Teasing" is a label for what is regarded as aggressive actions in this community.

7. Heil and Macdonald (2008) might interpret this in a slightly different but not incompatible way when they say with reference to health affecting choices made by Wiradjuri and Ngiyampaa people that "Notions of the social self produce a strategic use of time which recognises that life-as contingent is the norm, and that the demands of sociality critical to the constitution of the self have to be negotiated as they present themselves" (31).

8. At the Aboriginal community of Hermannsburg, similar displays of fast and dangerous driving are described a "making the car angry" (Austin-Broos 1996:15).

9. M. Tonkinson (1988) details sources of friction and inequality in relationships between Aboriginal and white women on the "Australian Frontier."

10. Peterson (1993) says: "The giving of care, nourishment, protection, and support is the foundation for an extensive and highly personal system of reciprocal responsibilities, rights, and commitments on which the right to make claims and demands is founded" (869).

11. "Blackfella business," unpackaged as "sorcery" and "cursing," was reported by the majority of respondents as a source of "feeling unsafe" according to a survey conducted at Ngukurr in the late 1990s (Taylor et al. 2000:96).

Conclusion

1. I have, in the past, argued that aggressive interactions at Numbulwar, though frequent, are for the most part acts of culturally structured aggression, that is, behavior that is expected and governed by norms that are usually successful in protecting victims from serious harm. In my book *Fighting Women* (Burbank 1994), I assessed Numbulwar in terms of three circumstances associated with greater violence against women in Aboriginal communities (Bolger 1991). These are: alcohol abuse, large heterogeneous communities composed of various language groups, and "cultural breakdown, dislocation, alienation and poverty" (16–18). What may be an increase in more injurious and less regulated violence, e.g., the severe beating of a woman by her intoxicated husband, could reflect changes in the first and third of these factors. Numbulwar remains a relatively homogeneous community.

2. For example, Wyrwoll et al. (2006) conclude a paper discussing the diet of rats experimentally stressed *in utero* with the following:

   The key finding of this study was that postnatal hyperleptinemia and hypertension [physiological states associated with ill health] programmed by excess glucocorticoid exposure *in utero* were completely prevented by a postnatal diet rich in n-3 fatty acids. In the absence of this dietary manipulation, programmed hyperleptinemia became fully apparent in both sexes by 6 months of age and was paralleled by changes in adipose expression of leptin mRNA. (604)

3. Shore (n.d.), contrasts attachment experiences of children in Samoa, Japan, and the United States, and suggests that such experiences are different because they take place in different cultural environments. The transformation of felt security—the ideal feeling state at the reunion of caretaker and child—varies, becoming the basis of different emotions, e.g.: *alofa* in Samoa, *amae* in Japan, and *love* in the Western experience (see also Hinton 1999:309–13). *Alofa, amae,* and *love* cannot be direct translations of one another, nor can any of them be reduced to "felt security." Nevertheless, felt security is an essential ingredient for their development.

4. Such evidence is also to be found in the bodies of most women. Natural selection's solution to the "obstetric dilemma" is a compromised human female physiology imposed by the incompatibilities of bipedalism, vaginal delivery, and a large fetal brain. The very tight fit of a baby's head in the birth canal's opening and the fact that generally our babies are born facing toward their mother's buttocks rather than *mons veneris* mean that our prehuman predecessors, and women today, would be likely to injure or kill their own infant were they to deliver it alone. This is not to say that it is impossible for women to deliver their own babies alone,

they sometimes do. For example, !Kung women aspire to the ideal of giving birth unassisted. Nevertheless, they may be criticized by their kin if they succeed in doing so (Shostak 1981:181). Natural selection is conceptualized as a slow process, the results of which are not perfect organisms, but those whose ancestors were more able than their conspecifics to leave descendants. It is not the fact that women may successfully give birth alone, but the greater probability that doing so will lead to their own or their child's injury and death that has, according to evolutionary arguments, given greater reproductive success to females who were usually delivered by others. It is for this reason that Trevathan and McKenna (1994) describe human parturition as a necessary "social event" (91).

Not only were others required to aid in the delivery of our ancestors' offspring, our babies' extreme immaturity and helplessness—another apparent result of the obstetric dilemma—have long required group assistance, in this case to support mothers and their dependent children for the many years it takes children to reach maturity (Lancaster and Lancaster 1987). This is not to assume the presence of a "nuclear family." There are many ways to be a "cooperative breeder" (Hrdy 2003; 2009). Individuals may be assisted by kin such as parents or siblings or, as is common in affluent Western populations, by stranger specialists, e.g., obstetricians, nannies, maternity hospitals, and childcare center staff. The three million–five million year existence of this hominid social event and our species' characteristic of "cooperative breeding" strongly implicate some form of social group as an environmental constant in our species' evolution.

References

Abbie, A. A. 1976 *The original Australians*. Sydney: Rigby.

ABS (Australian Bureau of Statistics) 2003 The health and welfare of Australia's Aboriginal and Torres Strait Islander peoples. Canberra: ABS.

—— 2005 The health and welfare of Australia's Aboriginal and Torres Strait Islander peoples, 2005. http://www.abs.gov.au/anstats/abs@nsf/Latestproducts/1256DAFA7B8DFOAACA2.

—— 2009 Discussion paper: Assessment of methods for developing life table for Aboriginal and Torres Strait Islander Australians, 2006. Canberra: ABS.

Abu-Lughod, Lila 1991 Writing against culture. In *Recapturing anthropology: Working in the present*, ed. R. Fox, pp. 137–62. Santa Fe: School of American Research Press.

Abu-Lughod, Lila and Catherine Lutz 1990 Introduction: Emotion, discourse, and the politics of everyday life. In *Language and the politics of emotion*, eds. C. Lutz and L. Abu-Lughod, pp. 1–23. Cambridge: Cambridge University Press.

Acciaioli, Gregory 1981 Knowing what you're doing: A review of Pierre Bourdieu's *Outline of a theory of practice*. *Canberra Anthropology* 4 (1): 23–51.

Adair, Linda and Andrew Prentice 2004 A critical evaluation of the foetal origins hypothesis and its implications for developing countries. *Nutrition* 143: 191–3.

Adelson, Naomi 2008 Discourses of stress, social inequities, and the everyday worlds of First Nations women in a remote northern Canadian community. *Ethos* 36 (3): 316–33.

Agar, Michael 2003 The story of crack: Towards a theory of illicit drug trends. *Addiction Research and Theory* 11 (1): 3–29.

Agar, Michael and Heather Reisinger 2001 Open marginality: Heroin epidemics in different groups. *Journal of Drug Issues* 31(3): 729–46.

Altman, J. C. 1984 Hunter-gatherer subsistence production in Arnhem Land: The original affluence hypothesis re-examined. *Mankind* 14 (3): 179–90.

—— 1987 *Hunter-gatherers today: An Aboriginal economy in north Australia*. Canberra: Australian Institute of Aboriginal Studies.

Altman, J. C. and Nicholas Peterson 1988 Rights to game and right to cash among contemporary Australian hunter-gatherers. In *Hunters and gatherers 2: Property, power and ideology*, eds. T. Ingold, D. Riches, and J. Woodburn, pp. 75–94. Oxford: Berg.

Anderson, Ian 2007 Understanding the process. In *Social determinants of Indigenous health*, eds. B. Carson, T. Dunbar, R. Chenhall, and R. Bailie, pp. 21–40. Crows Nest, NSW: Allen and Unwin.

Austin-Broos, Diane 1996 "Two Laws," ontologies, histories: Ways of being Aranda today. *The Australian Journal of Anthropology* 7 (1): 1–20.

——— 2003 Places, practices, and things: The articulation of Arrente kinship with welfare and work. *American Ethnologist* 30 (1): 118–35.

——— 2009 *Arrente present, Arrente past: Invasion, violence, and imagination in Indigenous Central Australia*. Chicago: University of Chicago Press.

Bailie, Ross 2007 Housing. In *Social determinants of Indigenous health*, eds. B. Carson, T. Dunbar, R. Chenhall, and R. Bailie, pp. 203–30. Crows Nest, NSW: Allen and Unwin.

Barber, Marcus 2008 A place to rest: Dying, residence and community stability in remote Arnhem Land. In *Mortality, mourning and mortuary practices in Indigenous Australia*, eds. K. Glaskin, M. Tonkinson, Y. Musharbash, and V. Burbank, pp. 153–69. London: Ashgate.

Barker, David 1994 *Mothers, babies, and disease in later life*. London: BMJ Publishing.

——— 2004 The developmental origins of chronic adult disease. *Acta Paediatric Supp.* 1 446: 26–33.

Barry, Herbert, Irvin Child, and Margaret Bacon 1959 Relations of child training to subsistence economy. *American Anthropologist* 61: 51–63.

Bateson, Gregory 1972 *Steps to an ecology of mind*. New York: Ballantine Books.

Bateson, Patrick and Paul Martin 2000 *Design for a life: How behaviour develops*. London: Vintage.

Bauer, F. H. 1964 *Historical geography of white settlement in part of northern Australia, Part 2, the Katherine-Darwin region*. Canberra: Industrial Research Organization.

Bayton, John 1965 *Cross over Carpentaria: Being a history of the Church of England in Northern Australia from 1865–1965*. Brisbane: W. R. Smith and Paterson.

Beck, Eduard 1985 *The enigma of Aboriginal health: Interaction between biological, social and economic factors in Alice Springs town-camps*. Canberra: Australian Institute of Aboriginal Studies.

Beckett, Jeremy 1996 Against Nostalgia: Place and memory in Myles Lalor's "oral history." *Oceania* 66 (4): 312–22.

Bentley, Gillain 1985 Hunter-gatherer energetics and fertility: A reassessment of the !Kung San. *Human Ecology* 13 (1): 79–109.

Bentley, Gillian, Richard Paine, and Jesper Boldsen 2001 Fertility changes with the prehistoric transition to agriculture: Perspectives from reproductive ecology and aleodemography. In *Reproductive ecology and human evolution*, ed. P. Ellison, pp. 203–31. New York: Aldine de Gruyter.

Bentley, Gillian, Tony Goldberg, and Grażyna Jasieńska 1993 The fertility of agricultural and non-agricultural traditional societies. *Population Studies* 47: 269–81.

Berndt, Catherine 1978 In Aboriginal Australia. In *Learning non-aggression: The experience of non-literate societies*, ed. A. Montagu, pp. 144–60. Oxford: Oxford University Press.

Berndt, Ronald 1977 Aboriginal identity: Reality or mirage. In *Aborigines and change: Australia in the '70s*, ed. R. Berndt, pp. 1–12. Canberra: Australian Institute of Aboriginal Studies.

Berndt, Ronald and Catherine Berndt 1964 *The world of the first Australians*. Sydney: Ure Smith.

Betzig, Laura 1989 Causes of conjugal dissolution: A cross-cultural study. *Current Anthropology* 30 (5): 654–76.

Biernoff, David 1979 Traditional and contemporary structures and settlement in eastern Arnhem land with particular reference to the Nunggubuyu. In *A Black reality: Aboriginal camps and housing in remote Australia*, ed. M. Heppell, pp. 153–79. Canberra: Australian Institute of Aboriginal Studies.

Birdsall, Christina 1988 All one family. In *Being Black: Aboriginal cultures in "settled" Australia*, ed. I. Keen, pp. 137–58. Canberra: Aboriginal Studies Press.

Boehm, Christopher 2004 Large-game hunting and the evolution of human sociality. In *The origins and nature of sociality*, eds. R. Sussman and A. Shapman, pp. 270–87. New York: Aldine de Gruyter.

Bolger, Audrey 1991 *Aboriginal women and violence*. Darwin: Australian National University, North Australian Research Unit.

Bourgois, Philippe 2003 Crack and the political economy of social suffering. *Addiction Research and Theory* 11 (2): 31–7.

Bowlby, John 1969 *Attachment. Attachment and loss*, Volume I. New York: Basic Books.

——— 1980 *Loss: Sadness and depression. Attachment and loss*, Volume III. New York: Basic Books.

Boyd, Robert and Peter Richerson 2008 Gene-culture coevolution and the evolution of social institutions. In *The Strungmann Forum report: Better than conscious? Decision making, the human mind, and implication for institutions*, eds. C. Engel and W. Singer, pp. 305–23. Cambridge, MA: MIT Press.

Boyer, Pascal 1993 Cognitive aspects of religious symbolism. In *Cognitive aspects of religious symbolism*, ed. P. Boyer, pp. 4–47. Cambridge: Cambridge University Press.

Boyer, Pascal and H. Clark Barrett 2005 Domain specificity and intuitive ontology. In *The handbook of evolutionary psychology*, ed. D. Buss, pp. 96–118. New York: John Wiley and Sons.

Brady, Kathleen and Rajita Sinha 2005 Co-occurring mental and substance use disorders: The neurobiological effects of chronic stress. *American Journal of Psychiatry* 162 (8): 1483–93.

Brady, Maggie 1992 *Heavy metal: The social meaning of petrol sniffing in Australia.* Canberra: Aboriginal Studies Press.

—— 1995 Broadening the base of interventions for Aboriginal people with alcohol problems. Technical Report No. 29. Sydney: University of NSW National Drug and Alcohol Research Centre.

Bräuer, Juliane, Josep Call, and Michael Tomasello 2006 Are apes really inequity averse? *Proceeding of the Royal Society B* 273: 3123–8.

Bretherton, Inge 1985 Attachment theory: Retrospect and prospect. In *Growing points of attachment theory and research*, eds. I. Bretherton and E. Waters, pp. 3–38. Monographs of the Society for Research in Child Development Serial Number 309: 50: 1–2.

Brown, Ryan, Nancy Adler, Carol Worthman, William Copeland, Jane Costello, and Adrian Angold 2008 Cultural and community determinants of subjective social status among Cherokee and White youth. *Ethnicity and Health* 13 (4): 289–303.

Brunner, Eric and David Marmot 1999 Social organization, stress and health. In *Social determinants of health*, eds. E. Brunner and D. Marmot, pp. 17–23 Oxford: Oxford University Press.

Burbank, Victoria 1980 Expressions of Anger and Aggression in an Australian Aboriginal Community. PhD dissertation, Rutgers University, New Brunswick, NJ.

—— 1985 Mirriri as ritualized aggression. *Oceania* 56: 47–55.

——1988 *Aboriginal adolescence: Maidenhood in an Australian community.* New Brunswick: Rutgers University Press.

—— 1994 *Fighting women: Anger and aggression in Aboriginal Australia.* Berkeley: University of California Press.

—— 1999 Fight! fight!: Men, women and interpersonal aggression in an Australian Aboriginal community. In *To have and to hit: Cultural perspectives on wife beating*, 2nd ed., eds. D. Counts, J. Brown, and J. Campbell, pp. 43–52. Chicago: University of Illinois Press.

—— 2000 "The lust to kill" and the Arnhem Land sorcerer: An exercise in integrative anthropology. *Ethos* 28 (3): 410–44.

—— 2006 From bedtime to on time: Why many Aboriginal people don't especially like participating in Western institutions. *Anthropological Forum* 16 (1): 3–20.

Burbank, Victoria and James Chisholm 1989 Old and new inequalities in a southeast Arnhem Land community: Polygyny, marriage age and birth spacing. In *Emergent inequalities in Aboriginal Australia*, ed. J. Altman, pp. 85–94. Oceania Monograph 38. Sydney: University of Sydney.

—— 1992 Gender differences in the perception of ideal family size in an Australian Aboriginal community. In *Father-child relations: Cultural and biosocial contexts*, ed. B. Hewlett, pp. 177–89. New York: Aldine de Gruyter.

—— 1998 Adolescent pregnancy and parenthood in an Australian Aboriginal community. In *Adolescence in the Pacific*, eds. G. Herdt and S. Leavitt, pp. 55–70. University of Pittsburgh Press: ASAO Series.

Burbank, Victoria, Katie Glaskin, Yasmine Musharbash, and Myrna Tonkinson 2008 Introduction: Indigenous ways of death in Australia, In *Mortality, mourning and mortuary practices in Indigenous Australia*, eds. K. Glaskin, M. Tonkinson, Y. Musharbash, and V. Burbank, pp. 1–20. London: Ashgate.

Campbell, Judy 1997 Smallpox in Aboriginal Australia, 1829–1831. In *Biological consequences of European expansion 1450–1800*, eds. K. Kiple and S. Beck, pp. 275–95. London: Ashgate.

Carson, Bronwyn, Terry Dunbar, Richard Chenhall, and Ross Bailie (eds.) 2007 *Social determinants of Indigenous health*. Crows Nest, NSW: Allen and Unwin.

Cawte, John 1978 Gross stress in small islands: A study in macropsychiatry. In *Extinction and survival in human populations*, eds. C. Laughlin, and I. Brady, pp. 95–121. New York: Columbia University Press.

Chisholm, James 1993 Death, hope and sex: Life history theory and the development of alternative reproductive strategies. *Current Anthropology* 34: 1–24.

——— 1999 *Death, hope and sex: Steps to an evolutionary ecology of mind and morality*. Cambridge: Cambridge University Press.

Chisholm, James and Victoria Burbank 1991 Monogamy and polygyny in southeast Arnhem Land: Male coercion and female choice. *Ethology and Socio-biology* 12: 291–313.

Cole, Keith 1977 A critical appraisal of Anglican mission policy and practice in Arnhem Land, 1908–1939. In *Aborigines and change: Australia in the '70s*. ed. R. Berndt, pp. 177–98. Canberra: Australian Institute of Aboriginal Studies.

——— 1979 *The Aborigines of Arnhem Land*. Adelaide: Rigby.

——— 1982 *A history of Numbulwar*. Bendigo, VIC: Keith Cole Publication.

——— 1985 *From mission to church: The CMS mission to the Aborigines of Arnhem land 1908–1985*. Bendigo, VIC: Keith Cole Publications.

Condon, John, Tony Barnes, Joan Cunningham, and Len Smith 2004 Improvements in Indigenous mortality in the Northern Territory over four decades. *Australian and New Zealand Journal of Public Health* 28 (5): 445–51.

Cowlishaw, Gillian 1981 The determinants of fertility among Australian Aborigines. *Mankind* 13 (1): 37–55.

——— 1982 Socialisation and subordination among Australian Aborigines. *Man* 17 (2): 492–507.

——— 1988 *Black, white or brindle: Race in rural Australia*. Cambridge: Cambridge University Press.

——— 2004 *Blackfellas, whitefellas and the hidden injuries of race*. Oxford: Blackwell Publishing.

Cox, Leonie 2009 Queensland Aborigines, multiple realities and the social sources of suffering: Psychiatry and moral regions of being. *Oceania* 79 (2): 97–120.

Coyne, James and Geraldine Downey 1991 Social factors and psychopathology: Stress, social support, and coping processes. *Annual Review of Psychology* 42: 401–25.

Cunningham, Joan and Yin Paradies 2000 Mortality of Aboriginal and Torres Strait Islander Australians 1997. Occasional Paper, Australian Bureau of Statistics: Canberra.

Damasio, Antonio 2003 Feelings of emotion and the self. *Annals of the New York Academy of Science* 1001: 253–61.

D'Andrade, Roy 1992 Schemas and motivation. In *Human motives and cultural models*, eds. R. D'Andrade and C. Strauss, pp. 23–44. Cambridge: Cambridge University Press.

——— 1995 *The development of cognitive anthropology*. Cambridge: Cambridge University Press.

Demakakos, Panayotes, James Nazroos, Elizabeth Breeze, and Michael Marmot 2008 Socioeconomic status and health: The role of subjective social status. *Social Science and Medicine* 67: 330–40.

Dollard, John. Leonard Doob, Neal Miller, O. H. Mowrer, and Robert Sears 1969 (1939) *Frustration and aggression*. New Haven: Yale University Press.

Drake, A. J. and B. R. Walker 2004 The intergenerational effects of foetal programming: Non-genomic mechanisms for the inheritance of low birth weight and cardiovascular risk. *Journal of Endocrinology* 180: 1–16.

Draper, Patricia 2007 Conducting cross-cultural research in teams and the search for the "culture-proof" variable. *Menopause* 14 (4): 680–7.

Dressler, William 1990 Lifestyle, stress and blood pressure in a Southern Black community. *Psychosomatic Medicine* 52: 182–98.

——— 1991a Social support, lifestyle incongruity, and arterial blood pressure in a Southern Black community. *Psychosomatic Medicine* 53: 608–20.

——— 1991b *Stress and adaptation in the context of culture: Depression in a Southern Black community*. Albany: State University of New York Press.

Dressler, William, Kathryn Oths, and Clarence Gravlee 2005 Race and ethnicity in public health research: Models to explain health disparities. *Annual Review of Anthropology* 2005: 231–52.

Driessen, Henk 1999 Comments. *Current Anthropology* 40 (4): 431–2.

Dumont, Louis 1970 *Homo hierarchicus: The caste system and its implications*. London: Weidenfeld and Nicholson.

Durkheim, Emile 1965 (1915) *The elementary forms of the religious life*. New York: The Free Press.

Eades, Diane 1993 Language and the law: White Australia v Nancy. In *Language and culture in Aboriginal Australia,* eds. M. Walsh and C. Yallop, pp. 181–90. Canberra: Aboriginal Studies Press.

Eastwell, H. 1976 Associative illness among Aboriginals. *Australian and New Zealand Journal of Psychiatry* 10: 89–94.

Eisenberger, Naomi and Matthew Lieberman 2004 Why rejection hurts: A common neural alarm system for physical and social pain. *Trends in Cognitive Science* 8 (7): 294–300.

Ellison, Peter 2001 *On fertile ground*. Cambridge, MA: Harvard University Press.

———— 2005 Evolutionary perspectives on the foetal origins hypothesis. *American Journal of Human Biology* 17: 113–18.

Elman, Jeffrey, Elizabeth Bates, Mark Johnson, Annette Karmiloff-Smith, Domenico Parisi, and Kim Plunkett 1996 *Rethinking innateness: A connectionist perspective on development*. Cambridge: MIT Press.

Elzanowski, Andrzej 1993 The moral career of vertebrate values. In *Evolutionary ethics*, eds. M. Nitecki and D. Nitecki, pp. 259–74. New York: SUNY Press.

Ericksson, J. G., T. Forsen, J. Tuomilehto, C. Osmond, and D. J. P. Barker 2003 Early adiposity rebound in childhood and risk of type 2 diabetes in adult life. *Diabetologia* 10.1007/s00125–002–1012–5.

Erikson, Erik 1968 *Identity, youth and crisis*. New York: W. W. Norton.

Fajans, Jane 2006 Autonomy and relatedness: Emotions and the tension between individuality and sociality. *Critique of Anthropology* 26 (1): 103–19.

Fanon, Frantz 1967 *Black skin, white masks*. New York: Grove.

Farmer, Paul 2004 An anthropology of structural violence. *Current Anthropology* 45: 305–25.

Fehr, Ernst and Joseph Henrich 2003 Is strong reciprocity a maladaptation?: On the evolutionary foundations of human altruism. In *Genetic and cultural evolution of cooperation*, ed. P. Hammerstein, pp. 55–82. Cambridge, MA: MIT Press.

Fenichel, Otto 1945. *The psychoanalytic theory of neurosis*. New York: Norton.

Fernandez, James 1991 Introduction: Confluents of inquiry. In *Beyond metaphor: The theory of tropes in anthropology*, ed. J. Fernandez, pp. 1–16. Stanford: Stanford University Press.

Fessler, Daniel and Kevin Haley 2003 The strategy of affect: Emotions in human cooperation. In *Genetic and cultural evolution of cooperation*, ed. P. Hammerstein, pp. 7–36. Cambridge, MA: MIT Press.

Fiske, Alan 1992 The four elementary forms of sociality: Framework for a unified theory of social relations. *Psychological Review* 99 (4): 689–723.

Flinn, Mark, Carol Ward and Robert Noone 2005 Hormones and the human family. In *The handbook of evolutionary psychology*, ed. D. Buss, pp. 552–80. New York: John Wiley and Sons.

Frake, Charles 1994 Cognitive anthropology: An origin story. In *The making of psychological anthropology II*, eds. M. Suarez-Orozco, G. Spindler, and L. Spindler, pp. 244–53. Fort Worth: Harcourt Brace College Publishers.

Franklin, Margaret-Ann and Isobel White 1991 The history and politics of Aboriginal health. In *The health of Aboriginal Australia*, eds.

J. Reid and P. Trompf, pp. 1–36. Marrickville, NSW: Harcoutrt Brace Jovanovich Group (Australia) Pty Ltd.

Freud, Sigmund 1989 (1905) Fragment of an analysis of a case of hysteria ("Dora"). In *The Freud reader*, ed. P. Gay, pp. 172–238. New York: W. W. Norton and Company.

——— 1989 (1907) Obsessive action and religious practices. In *The Freud reader*, ed. P. Gay, pp. 429–36. New York: W. W. Norton and Company.

Geertz, Clifford 1973 *The interpretation of cultures: Selected essays by Clifford Geertz*. New York: Basic Books.

Gerrard, Grayson 1989 Everyone will be jealous for that mutika. *Mankind* 19 (2): 95–111.

Gilbert, Kevin 1978 *Living black: Blacks talk to Kevin Gilbert*. Ringwood, Victoria: Penguin.

Gilligan, Carol 1982 *In a different voice*. Cambridge, MA: Harvard University Press.

Glaskin, Katie, Myrna Tonkinson, Yasmine Musharbash, and Victoria Burbank (eds) 2008 *Mortality, mourning and mortuary practices in Indigenous Australia*. London: Ashgate.

Gluckman, Peter, Mark Hanson, and Alan Beedle 2007 Early life events and their consequences for later disease: A life history and evolutionary perspective. *American Journal of Human Biology* 19 (1): 1–19.

Goodenough, Ward 1971 Culture, language and society. Addison-Wesley Module in Anthropology No. 7, Reading, Mass: Addison-Wesley Publishing.

Grady, J. 1997 Foundations of meaning: Primary metaphors and primary scenes. PhD dissertation, University of California, Berkeley, CA.

Gray, M. C., B. H. Hunter, and J. Taylor 2004 *Health expenditure, income and health status among Indigenous and other Australians*. Canberra: ANU Press. http://.anu.edu.au/caepr_sereis/no/moblie-devices/index.html.

Greenfield, Susan 2000 *The private life of the brain: Emotions, consciousness and the secret of the self*. New York: Wiley.

Gregg, Gary 1998 Culture, personality and the multiplicity of identity: evidence from North African life narratives. *Ethos* 26 (2): 120–52.

Gunnar, Megan and Karina Quevedo 2007 The neurobiology of stress and development. *Annual Review of Psychology* 58: 145–73.

Hamilton, Annette 1981 *Nature and nurture: Aboriginal child-rearing in North-Central Arnhem Land*. Canberra: Australian Institute of Aboriginal Studies.

Hamilton, David and Robert Gifford 1976 Illusory correlation in interpersonal perception: A cognitive basis of stereotypic judgement. *Journal of Experimental Social Psychology* 12: 392–407.

Harding, J. E. 2001 The nutritional basis of the foetal origins of adult disease. *International Journal of Epidemiology* 30 (1): 15–23.

Harris, John 1993 Losing and gaining a language: The story of Kriol in the Northern Territory. In *Language and culture in Aboriginal Australia*, eds. M. Walsh and C. Yallop, pp. 145–54. Canberra: Aboriginal Studies Press.

Hausfeld, R. G. 1977 Basic value orientations: Change and stress in two Aboriginal communities. In *Aborigines and change: Australia in the '70s,* ed. R. Berndt, pp. 266–87. Canberra: Australian Institute of Aboriginal Studies.

Hazan, Cindy and Phillip Shaver 1987 Romantic love conceptualized as an attachment process. *Journal of Personality and Social Psychology* 52: 511–24.

Heath, Jeffrey 1978 *Linguistic diffusion in Arnhem Land.* Canberra: Australian Institute of Aboriginal Studies.

———— 1980 *Nunggubuyu myths and ethnographic texts.* Canberra: Australian Institute of Aboriginal Studies.

———— 1982 *Nunggubuyu dictionary.* Canberra: Australian Institute of Aboriginal Studies.

Heil, Daniela and Gaynor Macdonald 2008 "Tomorrow comes when tomorrow comes": Managing Aboriginal health within an ontology of life-as-contingent. *Oceania* 78 (3): 299–319.

Hendrix, Lewellyn 1985 Economy and child training reexamined. *Ethos* 13 (3): 246–61.

Hiatt, Les 1985 Maidens, males, and Marx: Some contrasts in the work of Frederick Rose and Claude Meillassoux. *Oceania* 56: 34–46.

Hinkson, Melinda 2005 The intercultural challenge of Stanners' first field-work. *Oceania* 75: 195–208.

Hinkson, Melinda and Benjamin Smith 2005 Introduction: Conceptual moves towards an intercultural analysis. *Oceania* 2005 (3): 157–66.

Hinton, Alex 1999 Outline of a bioculturally based, "processual" approach to the emotions. In *Biocultural approaches to the emotions,* ed. A. Hinton, pp. 299–328. Cambridge: Cambridge University Press.

Hirschfeld, Lawrence 1997 The conceptual politics of race: Lessons from our children. *Ethos* 25 (1): 65–92.

Hollan, Douglas 2008 Being there: On the imaginative aspects of under-standing others and being understood. *Ethos* 36 (4): 475–89.

Hollan, Douglas and C. Jason Throop 2008 Whatever happened to empa-thy?: Introduction. *Ethos: Special Issue: Whatever happened to empa-thy?* 36 (4): 385–401.

Howell, Nancy 1979 *Demography of the Dobe !Kung.* New York: Academic Press.

Hrdy, Sarah 2003 The optimal number of fathers: Evolution, demography, and history in the shaping of female mate preferences. In *Evolutionary psychology: Alternative approaches,* eds. S. Scher and F. Rauscher, pp. 111–33. Boston: Kluwer Academic Publishers.

Hrdy, Sarah 2009 *Mothers and others: The evolutionary origins of mutual understanding.* Cambridge, MA: Belknap Press of Harvard University Press.

Hughes, Earl 1971 *Nunggubuyu-English dictionary.* Oceania Linguistic Monographs, No 14. Sydney: University of Sidney.

Hunter, Ernest 1993 *Aboriginal health and history: Power and prejudice in remote Australia.* Cambridge: Cambridge University Press.

Huntington, Richard and Peter Metcalf 1979 *Celebrations of death: The anthropology of mortuary ritual.* Cambridge: Cambridge University Press.

Hutchins, Edwin 1987 Myth and experience in the Trobriand Islands. In *Cultural models in language and thought*, eds. D. Holland and N. Quinn, pp. 269–89. Cambridge: Cambridge University Press.

Jackman, M. R. and R. W. Jackman 1973 Interpretation of relation between objective and subjective social status. *American Sociological Review* 38 (5): 569–82.

Kakar, Sudhir 1996 *The colors of violence: cultural identities, religion and conflict.* Chicago: University of Chicago Press.

Kawachi, Ichiro and Bruce Kennedy 2002 *The health of nations: Why inequality is harmful for your health.* New York: The New Press.

Keen, Ian 1995 Metaphor and metalanguage: Groups in Northeast Arnhem Land. *American Ethnologist* 22 (3): 505–27.

———— 2000 A bundle of sticks: The debate over Yolngu clans. *Journal of the Royal Anthropological Institute* 6: 419–36.

Keesing, Roger 1974 Theories of culture. *Annual Review of Anthropology* 3: 73–97.

Khantzian, E. J. 1985 The self-medication hypothesis of addictive disorders: Focus on heroin and cocaine dependence. *American Journal of Psychiatry* 142: 1259–64.

Kirmayer, Laurence 2008 Empathy and alterity in cultural psychiatry. *Ethos* 36 (4): 457–74.

Kluckhohn, Florence and Fred Strodtbeck 1961 *Variations in value orientations.* New York: Row, Peterson.

Kövecses, Zoltán 2005 *Metaphor in culture: Universality and variation.* Cambridge: Cambridge University Press.

Kuzawa, Christopher 2005 Fetal origins of developmental plasticity: Are fetal cues reliable predictors of future nutritional environments. *American Journal of Human Biology* 17: 5–21.

Lakoff, George and Mark Johnson 1980 *Metaphors we live by.* Chicago: University of Chicago Press.

———— 1999 *Philosophy in the flesh: The embodied mind and its challenge to Western thought.* New York: Basic Books

Lancaster, Jane 1986 Human adolescence and reproduction: An evolutionary perspective. In *School-age pregnancy and parenthood: Biosocial dimensions*, eds. J. Lancaster and B. Hamburg, pp. 17–38. New York: Aldine de Gruyter.

Lancaster, Jane and Chet Lancaster 1987 The watershed: Change in parental-investment and family formation strategies in the course of human evolution. In *Parenting across the life span: Biosocial dimensions*, eds. J. Lancaster, J. Altmann A. Rossi, L. Sherrod, pp. 187–205. New York: Aldine de Gruyter.

Langton, Marcia 1993 *"Well, I heard it on the radio and I saw it on the television"...An essay for the Australian Film Commission on the politics and aesthetics of filmmaking by and about Aboriginal people and things.* Woolloomoolo, NSW: Australian Film Commission.

Lazarus, Richard 1999 *Stress and emotion: A new synthesis.* New York: Springer.

Lear, Jonathan 2006 *Radical hope: Ethics in the face of cultural devastation.* Cambridge, MA: Harvard University Press.

LeDoux, Joseph 1996 *The emotional brain: The mysterious underpinnings of emotional life.* New York: Simon and Schuster.

―――― 2002 *Synaptic self: How our brains become who we are.* New York: Viking.

LeVine, Robert 1973 *Culture, behavior and personality.* Chicago: Aldine.

Levinson, Stephen 2006 Introduction: The evolution of culture in a microcosm. In *Evolution and culture*, eds. S. Levinson and P. Jaisson, pp. 1–41. Cambridge, MA: MIT Press.

Linger, Daniel 1994 Has culture theory lost its minds? *Ethos* 22 (3): 284–315.

―――― 2005 *Anthropology through a double lens: Public and personal worlds in human theory.* Philadelphia: University of Pennsylvania Press.

Lutz, Catherine 1985 Ethnopsychology compared to what?: Explaining behaviour and consciousness among the Ifaluk. In *Person, self and experience: Exploring Pacific ethnopsychologies*, eds. G. White and J. Kirkpatrick, pp. 35–79. Berkeley: University of California Press.

―――― 1988 *Unnatural emotions: Everyday sentiments on a Micronesian atoll and their challenge to Western theory.* Chicago: University of Chicago Press.

Macdonald, Gaynor 1988 A Wiradjuri fight story. In *Being Black: Aboriginal culture in "settled" Australia*, ed. I. Keen, pp. 179–99. Canberra: Aboriginal Studies Press.

―――― 2001 Does "culture" have "history"? Thinking about continuity and change in central New South Wales. *Aboriginal History* 25: 176–99.

―――― 2008 "Promise me you'll come to my funeral": Putting a value on Wiradjuri life through death. In *Mortality, mourning and mortuary practices in Indigenous Australia*, eds. K. Glaskin, Y. Musharbash, M. Tonkinson, and V. Burbank, pp. 121–36. London: Ashgate.

Makkreel, Rudolf 1995 *Einfuhlung.* In *The Cambridge dictionary of philosophy*, ed. R. Audi, p. 219. Cambridge: Cambridge University Press.

Malinowski, Bronislaw 1948 *Magic, science and religion.* London: Faber and West.

Marcus, George and Michael Fischer 1986 *Anthropology as cultural critique: An experimental moment in the human sciences.* Chicago: Chicago University Press.

Marmot, Michael and Richard Wilkinson (eds.) 1999 *Social determinants of health*. Oxford: Oxford University Press.

Masson, E. 1913 Report on Roper River Mission. Unpublished report in Australian Archives.

McArthur, Margaret 1960 Food consumption and dietary levels of groups of Aborigines living on naturally occurring foods. In *Records of the Australian America scientific expedition* volume 2, ed. C. P. Mountford, pp. 90–135. Melbourne: Melbourne University Press.

McCullough, Megan 2008 "Poor black bastard can't shake-a-leg": Humour and laughter in urban Aboriginal North Queensland, Australia. *Anthropological Forum* 18 (3): 279–86.

McEwen, Bruce and John Wingfield 2003 The concept of allostasis in biology and biomedicine. *Hormones and Behaviour* 43: 2–15.

McGrath, Ann (ed.) 1995 *Contested ground: Australian Aborigines under the British Crown*. St. Leonards, NSW: Allen and Unwin.

McKnight, David 2005 *Of marriage, violence and sorcery: The quest for power in Northern Queensland*. London: Ashgate.

Mechanic, David 2007 Population health: Challenges for science and society. *The Milbank Quarterly* 85 (3): 533–59.

Memmi, Albert 1974 (1957) *The colonizer and the colonized*. London: Souvenir Press.

Mercer, John 1978 *Good morning lumbarra: Stories for children based upon the experiences of a missionary amongst Aborigines at Numbulwar in Arnhem Land, North Australia*. Mt Tamborine, Qld: Published by the author.

Merlan, Francesca 1978 "Making people quiet" in the pastoral north: Reminiscences of Elsey Station. *Aboriginal History* 2 (1): 70–105.

――― 1998 *Caging the rainbow: Places, politics and Aborigines in a North Australian town*. Honolulu: University of Hawaii Press.

――― 2005 Explorations towards intercultural accounts of socio-cultural reproduction and change. *Oceania* 75 (3): 167–82.

――― 2006 European settlement and the making and unmaking of Aboriginal identities. *The Australian Journal of Anthropology* 17 (2): 179–95.

Moffatt, Michael ND American friendship and the individual self. Unpublished manuscript.

Morphy, Howard and Frances Morphy 1984 The "myths" of Ngalakan history: Ideology and images of the past in Northern Australia. *Man* 19: 459–78.

Musharbash, Yasmine 2007 Boredom, time and modernity: An example from Aboriginal Australia. *American Anthropologist* 109 (2): 307–17.

――― 2008 *Yuendumu everyday. Contemporary life in remote Aboriginal Australia*. Canberra: Aboriginal Studies Press.

Myers, Fred 1980 The cultural basis of politics in Pintupi life. *Mankind* 12: 197–214.

—— 1986 *Pintupi country, Pintupi self: Sentiment, place, and politics among Western Desert Aborigines*. Washington: Smithsonian Institution Press.

—— 1988 Burning the truck and holding the country: Property, time, and the negotiation identity among Pintupi Aborigines. In *Hunters and gatherers 2: Property, power and ideology*, eds. T. Ingold, D. Riches, and J. Woodburn, pp. 52–74. Oxford: Berg.

Nguyen, Vinh-Kim and Karine Peschard 2003 Anthropology, inequality, and disease: A review. *Annual Review of Anthropology* 32: 447–74.

NTCF 2002 The Northern Territory curriculum framework. Darwin: Department of Employment, Education and Training.

Nussbaum, Martha 1995 Human capabilities: Female human beings. In *Women, culture and development: A study of human capabilities*, eds. M. Nussbaum and J. Glover, pp. 61–104. Oxford: Clarendon Press.

Obeyesekere, Gananath 1981 *Medusa's hair: An essay on personal symbols and religious experience*. Chicago: University of Chicago Press.

—— 1990 *The work of culture: Symbolic transformation in psychoanalysis and anthropology*. Chicago: University of Chicago Press.

O'Donnell, Rosemary 2007 The value of autonomy: Christianity, organisation and performance in an Aboriginal community. PhD dissertation, University of Sydney, Sydney, NSW.

Panksepp, Jaak 1998 *Affective neuroscience: The foundation of human and animal emotions*. Oxford: Oxford University Press.

Paradies, Yin 2006 Beyond black and white: Essentialism, hybridity and indigeneity. *Journal of Sociology* 42 (4): 355–67.

Pearson, Noel 2000 *Our right to take responsibility*. Cairns: Noel Pearson and Associates.

Peterson, Nicholas 1993 Demand sharing: Reciprocity and the pressure for generosity among foragers. *American Anthropologist* 95(4): 860–74.

Peterson, Nicholas and John Taylor 2003 The modernizing of the Indigenous domestic moral economy: Kinship, accumulation and household composition. *The Asian Pacific Journal of Anthropology* 4 (1 & 2): 105–22.

Pulver, Lisa, Elizabeth Harris, and John Waldon 2007 An overview of the existing knowledge on the social determinants of Indigenous health and well being in Australia and New Zealand. Report of the Adelaide International Symposium. Adelaide, SA.

Quartz, Steven 2003 Toward a developmental evolutionary psychology: Genes, development, and the evolution of the human cognitive architecture. In *Evolutionary psychology: Alternative approaches*, eds. S. Scher and F. Rauscher, pp. 185–210. Boston: Kluwer Academic Publishers.

Quinn, Naomi 2003 Cultural selves. *Annals of the New York Academy of Science* 1001: 145–76.

Quinn, Naomi (ed.) 2005a *Finding culture in talk: A collection of methods*. New York: Palgrave Macmillan.

Quinn, Naomi (ed.) 2005b Introduction. In *Finding culture in talk: A collection of methods*, ed. N. Quinn, pp. 1–34. New York: Palgrave Macmillan.

—— 2005c Universals of child rearing. *Anthropological Theory* 5 (4): 475–514.

—— 2006 The self. *Anthropological Theory* 6 (3): 362–84.

Reay, Marie 1949 Native thought in rural New South Wales. *Oceania* 20 (2): 89–118.

Reddy, William 1997 Against constructionism: The historical ethnography of emotions. *Current Anthropology* 38: 327–51.

—— 2001 *The navigation of feeling: A framework of the history of emotions*. Cambridge: Cambridge University Press.

Redmond, Anthony 2005 Strange relatives: Mutualities and dependencies between Aborigines and pastoralists in the Northern Kimberley. *Oceania* 75: 234–46.

Reid, G. 1990 *A picnic with the natives: Aboriginal-European relations in the Northern Territory to 1910*. Melbourne: Melbourne University Press.

Reid, Janice 1983 *Sorcerers and Healing Spirits*. Canberra: ANU Press.

Reid, Janice and D. Lupton 1991 Introduction. In *The health of Aboriginal Australia*, eds. J. Reid and P. Trompf, pp. xi–xxii. Sydney: Harcourt Brace Jovanovich.

Reser, Joseph 1979 A matter of control: Aboriginal housing circumstances in remote communities and settlements. In *A Black reality: Aboriginal camps and housing in remote Australia*, ed. M. Heppell, pp. 65–96. Canberra: Australian Institute of Aboriginal Studies.

Ribeiro, Saulo, Susan Kennedy, Yolanda Smith, Christian Stohler, and Jon-Kar Zubieta 2005 Interface of physical and emotional stress regulation though the endogenous opioid system and μ-opioid receptors. *Progress in Neuro-Psychopharmacology and Biological Psychiatry* 29: 1264–80.

Richerson, Peter and Robert Boyd 2005 *Not by genes alone: How culture transformed human evolution*. Chicago: University of Chicago Press.

Riphagen, Marianne 2008 Black or white: Or varying shades of grey? Indigenous Australian photo-media artists and the "making of" Aboriginality. *Australian Aboriginal Studies* (1): 78–89.

Robben, Antonius 2004 Death and anthropology: An introduction. In *Death, mourning, and burial: A cross-cultural reader*, ed. A. Robben, pp. 1–16. Oxford: Blackwell Publishing.

Robbins, Joel 2007 Between reproduction and freedom: Morality, value, and radical cultural change. *Ethnos* 72 (3): 293–314.

Rosaldo, Renato 1984 Grief and a headhunter's rage: On the cultural force of emotions. In *Play, text and story*, ed. E. Bruner. Proceedings of the 1983 Meeting of the American Ethnological Society. Washington, D.C.

Rumsey, Alan 2004 Ethnographic macro-tropes and anthropological theory. *Anthropological Theory* 4 (3): 267–98.

Russell, James 2003 Core affect and the psychological construction of emotion. *Psychological Review* 110 (1): 145–72.

Sackett, Lee 1978 Punishment as ritual: Man-making among Western Desert Aborigines. *Oceania* 49: 110–27.

Saggers, Sherry and Dennis Gray 1991 *Aboriginal health and society: The traditional and contemporary Aboriginal struggle for better health.* St. Leonards, NSW: Allen and Unwin Pty Ltd.

——— 2007 Defining what we mean. In *Social determinants of Indigenous health*, eds. B. Carson, T. Dunbar, R. Chenhall, and R. Bailie, pp. 1–20. Crows Nest, NSW: Allen and Unwin.

Sahlins, Marshall 2000 (1993) Goodbye to *tristes tropes*: Ethnography in the context of modern world history. In *Culture in practice: Selected essays*, ed. M. Sahlins, pp. 471–500. New York: Zone Books.

Sanders, William 2005 CDEP and ATSIC as bold experiments in governing differently: But where to now? In *Culture, economy and governance in Aboriginal Australia: Proceeding of a workshop of the Academy of the Social Sciences in Australia held at the University of Sydney 30 November–1 December, 2004*, eds. D. Austin-Broos and G. Macdonald, pp. 203–12. Sydney: Sydney University Press.

Sansom, Basil 1980 *The camp at Wallaby Cross: Aboriginal fringe dwellers in Darwin*. Canberra: Australian Institute of Aboriginal Studies.

——— 1988 A grammar of exchange. In *Being Black: Aboriginal cultures in "settled" Australia*, ed. I. Keen, pp. 159–77. Canberra: Australian Institute of Aboriginal and Torres Strait Islander Studies.

Sapolsky, Robert 1993 Endocrinology alfresco: Psychoendocrine studies of wild baboons. *Recent Progress in Hormone Research* 48: 437–68.

——— 2004 Social status and health in humans and other animals. *Annual Review of Anthropology* 33: 393–418.

Scheffler, Harold 1978 *Australian kin classification*. Cambridge: Cambridge University Press.

Scheper-Hughes, Nancy and Margaret Lock 1987 The mindful body: A prolegomenon to future work in medical anthropology. *Medical Anthropology Quarterly* 1: 6–41.

Seligman, Martin 1975 *Helplessness: On depression, development, and death*. San Francisco: W. H Freeman and Company.

Sen, Amartya. 1992 *Inequality re-examined*. Cambridge, MA: Harvard University Press.

Senior, Kate 2003 A gudbala laif? Health and wellbeing in a remote Aboriginal community—what are the problems and where lies responsibility? PhD dissertation, Australian National University, Canberra, ACT.

Sennett, Richard and Jonathan Cobb 1972 *The hidden injuries of class*. New York: W. W. Norton.

Shapiro, Warren 1979 *Social organization in Aboriginal Australia*. New York: St. Martin's Press.

——— 1981 *Miwuyt marriage: The cultural anthropology of affinity in Northeast Arnhem Land*. Philadelphia: ISHI.

Sharp, Lauriston 1952 Steel axes for Stone Age Australians. In *Human problems in technological change: A casebook*, ed. E. Spicer, pp. 446–60. New York: Wiley.

Shell-Duncan, Bettina and Stacie Yung 2004 The maternal depletion transition in northern Kenya: The effects of settlement, development and disparity. *Social Science and Medicine* 58: 2485–98.

Shore, Bradd 1988 Interpretation under fire. *Anthropological Quarterly* 61 (4): 161–78.

———— 1996 *Culture in mind: Cognition, culture, and the problem of meaning*. Oxford: Oxford University Press.

———— ND Feeling our way: Toward a bio-cultural model of emotion. Unpublished manuscript.

Shostak, Marjorie 1981 *Nisa: The life and words of a !Kung woman*. Cambridge, MA: Harvard University Press.

Shweder, Richard 1996 True Ethnography: The lore, the law, and the lure. In *Ethnography and human development: Context and meaning in social inquiry*, eds. R. Jessor, A. Colby, and R. Shweder, pp. 13–52. Chicago: University of Chicago Press.

Shweder, Richard and Edmund Bourne 1984 Does the concept of the person vary cross-culturally? In *Culture theory: Essays on mind, self and emotions*, eds. R. Shweder and R. LeVine, pp. 158–99. Cambridge: Cambridge University Press.

Shweder, Richard, Jacqueline Goodenow, Giyoo Hatano, Robert LeVine, Hazel Markus, and Peggy Miller 1998 The cultural psychology of development: One mind, many mentalities. In *Handbook of child psychology*, 5th ed., ed. W. Damon, pp. 865–937. New York: John Wiley.

Singer, Tania 2006 The neuronal basis and ontogeny of empathy and mind reading: Review of literature and implication for future research. *Neuroscience and Biobehavioral Reviews* 30: 855–63.

Sökefeld, Martin 1999 Debating self, identity, and culture in anthropology. *Current Anthropology* 40 (4): 417–47.

Spiro, Melford 1951 Culture and personality: The natural history of a false dichotomy. *Psychiatry* 14: 19–46.

———— 1958 *Children of the kibbutz*. New York: Schocken Books.

———— 1993 Is the Western conception of the self "peculiar" within the context of the world cultures? *Ethos* 21 (2): 10753.

Strauss, Claudia and Naomi Quinn 1994 A cognitive/cultural anthropology. In *Assessing cultural anthropology*, ed. R. Borofsky, pp. 284–9. New York: McGraw-Hill.

———— 1997 *A cognitive theory of cultural meaning*. Cambridge: Cambridge University Press.

Sturmer , John von 1981 Talking with Aborigines. *Australian Institute of Aboriginal Studies Newsletter* N.S. No 15. Canberra.

Sullivan, Harry. S. 1970 (1954) *The psychiatric interview*. New York: Norton.

Super, Charles and Sara Harkness 1986 The developmental niche: A conceptualization at the interface of child and culture. *International Journal of Behavioural Development* 9: 545–69.

Sutton, Peter 2009 *The politics of suffering: Indigenous Australia and the end of the liberal consensus.* Melbourne: Melbourne University Press.

Taussig, Michael 1980 *The devil and commodity fetishism in South America.* Chapel Hill: University of North Caroline Press.

Taylor, J., J. Bern, and K. A. Senior 2000 *Ngurkurr at the millennium: A baseline profile for social impact planning in South-East Arnhem Land. Centre for Aboriginal Economic Policy Research.* Research Monograph No. 18, Australian National University, Canberra.

Taylor, Shelly and Annette Stanton 2007 Coping resources, coping processes and mental health. *Annual Review of Clinical Psychology* 3: 377–401.

Thompson, Christopher, Holly Syddall, Ian Rodin, Clive Osmond, and David Barker. 2001 Birth weight and the risk of depressive disorder in later life. *British Journal of Psychiatry* 179: 450–5.

Thomson, Donald 1936 Interim general report of preliminary expedition to Arnhem Land, Northern Territory of Australia, 1935–1936. Australian Institute of Aboriginal Studies, Canberra.

——— 1983 *Donald Thomson in Arnhem Land.* South Yarra, VIC: Currey O'Neil.

Tonkinson, Myrna 1988 Sisterhood or Aboriginal servitude? Black women and White women on the Australian frontier. *Aboriginal History* 12 (1–2): 27–39.

——— 1990 Is it in the blood? Australian Aboriginal identity. In *Cultural identity and ethnicity in the Pacific,* eds. J. Linnekin and L. Poyer, pp. 191–218. Honolulu: University of Hawaii Press.

——— 2008 Solidarity in shared loss: Death-related observances among the Martu of the Western Desert. In *Mortality, mourning and mortuary practices in Indigenous Australia,* eds. K. Glaskin, Y. Musharbash, M. Tonkinson, and V. Burbank, pp. 37–54. London: Ashgate.

——— 2011 Being Mardu: Change and challenge for some Western Desert young people today. In *Growing up in Central Australia: New anthropological studies of Aboriginal childhood and adolescence,* ed. U. Eickelkamp. Oxford: Berghahn Press.

Tonkinson, Myrna and Robert Tonkinson 2008 Coping with imposed change in remote Aboriginal communities: Policy, values and the struggle for control. Paper presented at CASCA Conference, Ottawa, Canada.

Tonkinson, Robert 1978 *The Mardudjara Aborigines: Living the dream in Australia's desert.* New York: Holt Rinehart and Winston.

——— 2004 Spiritual prescription, social reality: Reflections on religious dynamism. *Anthropological Forum* 14 (2): 183–201.

——— 2007a The Mardu Aborigines; On the road to somewhere. In *Globalization and changes in fifteen cultures: Born in one world, living in another*, eds. G. Spindler and J. Stockard, pp. 225–55. Belmont, CA: Thomson Wadsworth.

———— 2007b Aboriginal "difference" and "autonomy" then and now: Four decades of change in an eastern Desert Society. *Anthropological Forum* 17 (1): 41–60.

Trevathan, Wenda and James McKenna 1994 Evolutionary environments of human birth and infancy: Insights to apply to contemporary life. *Children's Environments* 11 (2): 88–104.

Trigger, David 1992 *Whitefella comin': Aboriginal responses to colonialism in northern Australia*. Cambridge: Cambridge University Press.

Trouillot, Michel-Rolph 2003 *Global transformations: Anthropology and the modern world*. New York: Palgrave Macmillan.

Turner, David 1974 *Tradition and transformation: A study of Aborigines in the Groote Eylandt area, northern Australia*. Canberra: Australian Institute of Aboriginal Studies.

Veblen, Thorstein 1918 *The theory of the leisure class*. New York: BW Huebsch.

Vogt, Evon and Ethel Albert 1966a The "comparative study of values in five cultures" project. In *People of Rimrock: A study of values in five cultures*, eds. E. Vogt and E. Albert, pp. 1–33. Cambridge, MA: Harvard University Press.

———— (eds.) 1966b *People of Rimrock: A study of values in five cultures*. Cambridge, MA: Harvard University Press.

Wahlbeck, Kristian, Tom Forsen, Clive Osmond, David Barker, and Johan Eriksson 2001 Association of schizophrenia with low maternal body mass index, small size at birth, and thinness during childhood. *Archives of General Psychiatry* Jan 58 (1): 48–52.

Wallace, Anthony 1961 *Culture fand personality*. New York: Random House.

Walsh, Michael 1993 Languages and their status in Aboriginal Australia. In *Language and culture in Aboriginal Australia*, eds. M. Walsh and C. Yallop, pp. 1–14. Canberra: Aboriginal Studies Press.

Warner, W. Lloyd 1937 *A Black civilization*. New York: Harper.

Westen, Drew and Glen Gabbard 2002a Developments in cognitive neuroscience: I. Conflict, compromise, and connectionism. *Journal of the American Psychoanalytic Association* 50: 54–98.

———— 2002b Developments in cognitive neuroscience: II. Implications for theories of transference. *Journal of the American Psychoanalytic Association* 50: 99–133.

Wharton, Edith 1966 *The house of mirth*. London: Constable.

Wierzbicka, Anna 1993 A conceptual basis for cultural psychology. *Ethos* 21 (2): 205–31.

———— 1996 *Semantics: Primes and universals*. Oxford: Oxford University Press.

———— 1999 *Emotion across languages and cultures: Diversity and universals*. Cambridge: Cambridge University Press.

—— 2005 Empirical universals of language as a basis for the study of other human universals and as a tool for exploring cross-cultural differences. *Ethos* 33 (2): 256–91.

Wilkinson, Richard 1996 *Unhealthy societies: The inflictions of inequality.* London: Routledge.

Worthman, Carol 1999 Evolutionary perspectives on the onset of puberty. In *Evolutionary Medicine*, eds. W. Trevathan, E. O. Smith, and J. McKenna, pp 135–63. Oxford: Oxford University Press.

Worthman, Carol and Jennifer Kuzara 2005 Life history and the early origins of health differentials. *American Journal of Human Biology* 17: 95–112.

Wyrwoll, Caitlin, Peter Mark, Trevor Mori, Ian Puddey, and Brendan Waddell 2006 Prevention of programmed hyperleptinemia and hypertension by postnatal dietary ω-3 Fatty Acids. *Endocrinology* 147 (1): 599–606.

Young, Elspeth 1981 *Tribal communities in rural areas: The Aboriginal component in the Australian economy.* Development Studies Centre, ANU, Canberra.

Zhao, Yuejen and Karen Dempsey 2006 Causes of inequality in life expectancy between Indigenous and non-Indigenous people in the Northern Territory, 1981–2000: A decomposition analysis. *Medical Journal of Australia* 184 (10): 490–4.

Index

CPSIA information can be obtained at www.ICGtesting.com
Printed in the USA
LVOW101934040112

262463LV00004B/1/P